A Dynamic Materia Medica of the Noble Gases

NEON

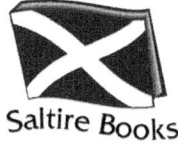
Saltire Books   *Saltire Books Limited, Glasgow, Scotland*

A Dynamic Materia Medica of the Noble Gases

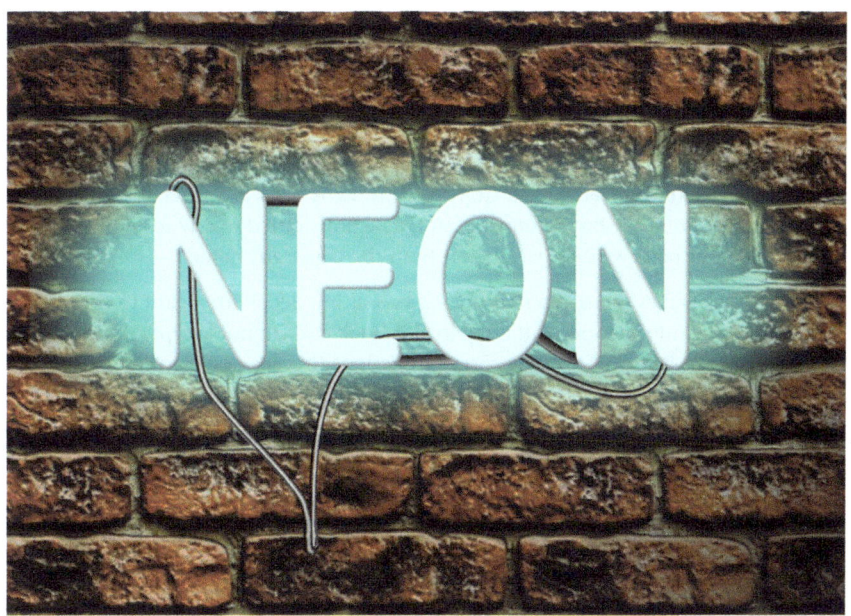

Jeremy Sherr

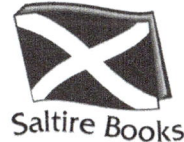
Saltire Books

Saltire Books Limited, Glasgow, Scotland

Published by Saltire Books Ltd

18–20 Main Street, Busby, Glasgow G76 8DU, Scotland
books@saltirebooks.com www.saltirebooks.com

Cover, Design, Layout and Text © Saltire Books Ltd 2016

 is a registered trademark

First published in 2016

Typeset by Type Study, Scarborough, UK in 9¼ on 13½ Stone Serif
Printed and bound in the UK by TJ International Ltd, Padstow

ISBN 978-1-908127-07-5

For Saltire
Project Development: Lee Kayne
Editorial: Steven Kayne
Designer: Phil Barker
Illustrator: Matt Canning
Additional graphics produced by Brenda Brown (brenda@brendapix.com)

CONTENTS

This book is dedicated to my beautiful son Louis:
May the force be with you

We are all in the gutter, but some of us are looking at the stars.

Oscar Wilde[i]

Some part of our being knows this is where we came from. We long to return. And we can. Because the cosmos is also within us. We're made of star-stuff. We are a way for the cosmos to know itself.

Carl Sagan[ii]

When the Holy One, Blessed Be He, created the world, He created seven firmaments above, created seven lands below, seven seas, seven rivers, seven days, seven weeks, seven years, seven times, seven thousand years that the world exists, that he sustained for six thousand years, and one thousand destroyed. And the Holy One, Blessed Be He, is in the seventh of them all.

Zohar[iii]

[i] Oscar Wilde: *Lady Windermere's Fan*. Available online at: http://www.goodreads.com/quotes/25-we-are-all-in-the-gutter-but-some-of-us

[ii] Carl Sagan: *Cosmos: A Personal Voyage. Episode 1*. Available online at: http://www.goodreads.com/quotes/413897-the-surface-of-the-earth-is-the-shore-of-the

[iii] Zohar: Matt DC (trans). *Zohar*: Pritzker Edition (6 vols.). Stanford, CA: Stanford University Press, 2004–2011.

ACKNOWLEDGMENTS

To all my dedicated friends and colleagues who have made this book possible. Materia medica is a group creation, 'As If One Person'. Thank you one and all.

To Silvie Gowan for her wonderful proving. Silvie is the MM potency of provings.

To Dynamis students 1993 for their proving of Neon.

To Wenda O'Reilly and California provers.

To John Morgan and Helios Pharmacy for preparing the remedy.

To Vivien Freund, Naomi Jones and Rebecca Stirrup for excellent editing and advising while volunteering to work alongside us in Homoeopathy for Health in Africa. Special thanks to Rebecca who had the guts to make me re-write several sections.

To Tina Quirk, who has been my friend, editor and proof-reader for many years, and has always helped make my work more readable and professional.

To Rafi Neu for help in evaluating this work, and for being my faithful partner in creating the Q-Rep. To his daughter Alma for illustration.

To Liz Norman, for being the best practice manager in the world.

To my colleagues who helped with editing and by contributing cases: Mary Aspinwall, Shelly Been, Geoff Johnson, Lou Klein, Roberto Petrucci, Hazel Rank-Broadley, Maria Schmelzer-Schenkel and Matthias Strelow.

To Steven and Lee Kayne of Saltire Books for support and excellent publishing.

To Brenda Brown for translating my thoughts into her beautiful illustrations. You can find Brenda at www.webtoon.com

To Jessica Lloyd-Jones for permission to use pictures of her noble sculptures. Jessica's work can be seen at http://www.jessicalloyd-jones.com/page18.htm

To my teacher Yorik Verete for Mishna and Cabbala lessons.

To Misha Norland for Flammarion.

To Carlo U. Segre, Professor of Physics, Illinois Institute of Technology.

To my spiritual teacher Rabbi Yaakov Melamed.

To all the poets whose works I have cited and quotes I have quoted. All poems are by Jeremy Sherr unless indicated otherwise.

To my wife Camilla, who always lets the positive bubble to the surface.

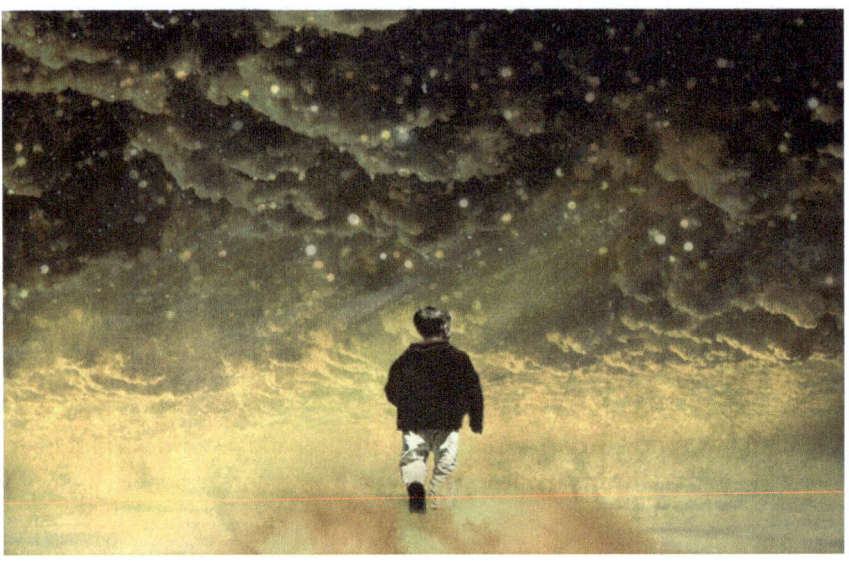

Illustration by Alma Neu

ABOUT THE AUTHOR

Jeremy Sherr has practised homoeopathy for over 30 years. He practises in London, New York and Tel Aviv and is Principal of The Dynamis School for Advanced Homoeopathic Medicine that offers one of the oldest post graduate courses in the world today. Jeremy has taught homoeopathy throughout the USA and Europe as well as in Canada, China, India, Mexico, Japan, Russia, South Africa, New Zealand and Australia. He has conducted 34 classical homoeopathic provings and is the author of *The Dynamics and Methodology of Homoeopathic Provings*, *Dynamic Provings Volumes I and II*, *Dynamic Materia Medica – Syphilis*, *Dynamic Materia Medica – Helium*, *Repertory of Mental Qualities* and *The Dynamic Case Taker*. He has published numerous articles on homoeopathy and has conducted several research programmes. Since 2008, Jeremy has been living in Tanzania. Together with his wife Camilla, he has established several rural clinics and is working in the local hospital. They have treated over 1500 AIDs patients and have established food programmes and a day care centre for children with AIDs.

ILLUSTRATION CREDITS

Cover page: Neon Sign by Brenda Brown www.webtoon.com

INTRODUCTION

It may be hard for an egg to turn into a bird: it would be a jolly sight harder for it to learn to fly while remaining an egg. We are like eggs at present. And you cannot go on indefinitely being just an ordinary, decent egg. We must be hatched or go bad.

C S Lewis[1]

Neon was my first proving from the noble gas series. It was 1993, and having studied the periodic table for some time, I decided to embark on the noble gas journey. I cannot recall why Neon was first. Perhaps it was about beginning something new, a new birth. Perhaps I was attracted by the neon signs that lit city centres. Maybe it was the line from the Simon and Garfunkel song playing in my head: *'And the people bowed and prayed, to the neon god they made'*.

I prepared and potentised this remedy myself. I travelled down to Helios Pharmacy, where my friend John Morgan and I bubbled neon gas through water for ten minutes. There is no perfect way to potentise a noble gas. Being inert, noble gases do not dissolve in water or mix with other chemicals, so I just had to trust the process. I recall my anxiety as I took one drop of the tincture and dissolved it in 99 drops of water. Could this really work? Would the transformation take place? As it turned out the amazing process of potentisation prevailed and a very distinct picture emerged from the proving. I remember Silvie's dismay when, after taking the first dose of the remedy, she opened her front door to find a load of discarded neon lights in her yard. Of course Silvie did not know the remedy substance as the experiment was double-blind.

While the original proving was conducted in England, a further proving was undertaken in California by Wenda O'Reilly, who was a Dynamis student at the time. Wenda later went on to expand her graduation project into a new translation and edition of the *Organon*. Perhaps this was one of the new births resulting from the Neon proving.[2]

As for myself, I experienced a strange feeling throughout the proving. I felt that I was trapped inside a 'cosmic egg'. The shell was about to crack, but it did not, and I was frustrated and impatient to find out what lay beyond the confines of this egg. I felt that someone was knocking on my shell, calling me to emerge, and I yearned to burst out into the new world that lay beyond, but I had no idea how to do this or where I was heading. I was beckoned by an unknown experience of which I had no concept.

Towards the end of the proving I was invited to a group meeting with a shaman. As this was a new experience for me I had no idea what to expect, but the man knocked on all of our doors and opened quite a few. For me it was a gateway to a whole new world. Until today, I do not really know what happened there, what changed, but something did.

The truth is that for many years I did not fully understand this remedy. Of course I comprehended the symptoms and perceived how they neatly fitted into a meaningful totality. I prescribed Neon successfully in several cases and lectured on the remedy many times. I recognised the way Neon fitted in with the other noble gases, how it dovetailed into the preceding and following periods, but the same strange feeling persisted: something was missing, something that would make the remedy come alive and make it complete. I had no idea what the missing element was, but I realised that the remedy picture as I understood it then was just too blissful to be clinically useful.

With this in mind, 18 years after the original proving, I began my re-investigation into the proving of element number 10, neon. I invite you to join me on this journey. To fully understand the ideas within it is important to read the first volume in this series of titles, *Dynamic Materia Medica – Helium* that contains an introduction to the Noble Gases.[3]

Jeremy Sherr,
November 2015

Reference

1   Lewis CS. Mere Christianity. In: *Broadcast Talks*. Norwich: The Canterbury Press, 1942. Available online at: http://www.brainyquote.com/quotes/quotes/c/cslewis131286.html

2   Hahnemann CS. *The Organon of the Healing Art* (6th edn). New Delhi: B Jain Publishers Pvt Ltd, 2003.

3   Sherr J. *Dynamic Materia Medica – Helium*. Glasgow: Saltire Books, 2013.

The full, re-edited and enhanced proving of Neon may be obtained at www.dynamis.edu

1

THE POTENCIES OF PERCEPTION

In this book I relate the 'levels of perception' of Neon with levels of potency. **This division into levels of potency is analogous to the level of our understanding and has nothing whatsoever to do with the potencies taken by the provers or to the potency one should prescribe in clinical cases.** The potency should be selected according to the totality of the case regardless of in which chapter the symptom lies.

We can roughly compare the study of neon, the element, to the mother tincture potency of perception, while the higher potencies of perception penetrate the innermost nature of the remedy's geometrical structure, metaphors and cosmic connotations.

The potencies and the corresponding levels of perception, ranging from the gross to the subtle, are as follows:

- The element itself represents purely chemical properties.
- The mother tincture represents the homoeopathic preparation as well as naturopathic or herbal use.
- The 12C represents physical affinities.
- The 30C represents general themes.
- The 200C represents essence, emotional pictures and signatures.
- The 1M and 10M potencies are an unravelling of the symptom configuration, a search for meaning in the totality. At these, and higher potencies, the precise words and expressions of provers become important. While the 1M further develops the emotional essence, the 10M explores the inner structure.
- The 50M represents subtle sensations and functions including the geometrical structure of the remedy.
- The CM explores the world of analogy and metaphor.
- The MM and beyond are an investigation into the esoteric roots of the remedy and the simple substance that lies beyond.[i]

---

[i] According to Kent, a follower of Swedenborg, simple substance is the spiritual essence and potential that lies within, behind and above the material world, It is the precursor of all events and material in the world, the energetic blueprint of life in all its varieties and manifestations.

According to my 'grammatical' method of analysis, the 12C and 30C represent nouns, the 200C and 1M are at the level of adjectives and adverbs, while the 50M represents verbs; movements in time and space.[1] The potencies beyond transcend grammar as they touch the language of poetry. Matching the remedy to the patient on the basis of the higher potencies of perception will yield deeper results; for optimum similarity, however, all levels should fit.

I do not intend the correspondence of potency levels to concepts to be precise or dogmatic; rather it is a general idea. Creating yet another table or system to which homoeopaths should rigidly adhere can only lead to problems.

Please note that the chapter titles refer to potencies of perception and are in no way related to potencies prescribed in cases. The potency prescribed in each case should be determined by the totality of the case, not by the chapter in which the symptom is presented.

I have placed the cases after the 50M chapter because most Neon cases can be solved using knowledge gained from the preceding levels of perception (12C to 50M). You can gain almost all you need to know about prescribing the remedy from these chapters. The higher-level chapters, CM and above, explore broader concepts rather than the individual remedy. Not everyone will feel comfortable with the information in these high-potency chapters. That is fine; there is no need to go there. I enjoy thinking of these things and maybe some readers will too.

Only a few selected quotes from the proving are cited in each section. It is important to read the proving as a whole to gain a thorough understanding of the remedy as many symptoms appear only in the complete proving document. The full proving can be obtained from www.dynamis.edu

When capitalised, Neon and other element names refer to homoeopathic remedies, while lower-case names such as neon refer to the basic elements. All original symptoms from the Neon proving are given as follows: Neon symptom. Some proving symptoms have been abbreviated or edited; however, the essential content has been preserved. The complete and original text can be found in the proving document itself. Keywords and phrases that I consider important are occasionally marked **in bold**.

Reference

1   Sherr J. *Dynamic Materia Medica – Syphilis: A Study of the Syphilitic Miasm* (2nd edn). Glasgow: Saltire Books, 2015.

2

NEON THE ELEMENT

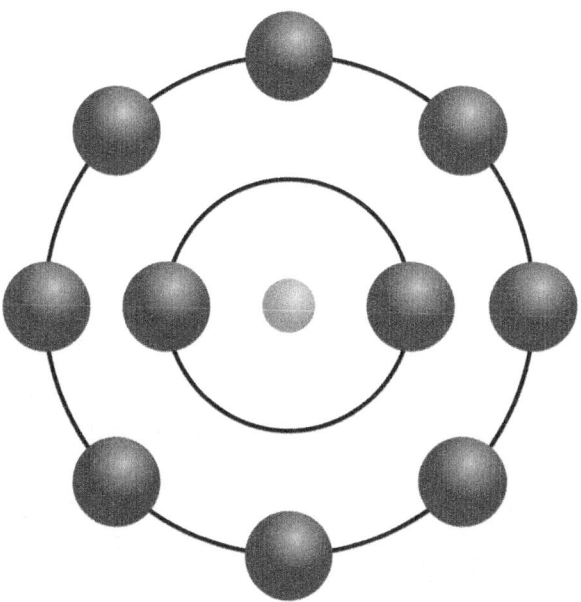

Figure 2.1 *Neon atom*

Neon has the symbol Ne, atomic number 10 and an atomic weight of 20.179. It is a colourless, odourless, noble gas. The name neon means 'new one'.

As an inert gas neon does not react with most substances but may form a compound with fluorine. Natural neon is a mixture of three isotopes. Six other unstable isotopes are known.

Neon is commercially extracted from air in which it is found in trace amounts. The gas freezes at minus 248.67 degrees Celsius so that when air is liquefied at minus 200 degrees Celsius, neon is left behind as a by-product. While neon makes up only 1 part per 65,000 of the earth's atmosphere, it is by mass the fifth most abundant element in the universe after hydrogen, helium, oxygen and carbon. Its rarity on Earth is due to its relative lightness, high vapour pressure at very low temperatures and chemical inertness, properties that keep it from being trapped in the condensing gas clouds that form around smaller planets such as Earth.

Neon originates in high-mass stars. It is created during the alpha process when helium is fused with oxygen. This process requires temperatures higher than 100 megakelvins and masses greater than 3 solar masses.

Neon was discovered in 1898 by British chemists Sir William Ramsay and Morris W. Travers while they were studying liquid air. They immediately noted the brilliant red colour that is emitted by gaseous neon when excited electrically.

Travers later wrote,

'... the blaze of crimson light from the tube told its own story and was a sight to dwell upon and never forget.'[1]

At ordinary voltages and currents neon has the most intense light discharge of all the rare gases. 'Neon' lights are made by sealing two electrodes within

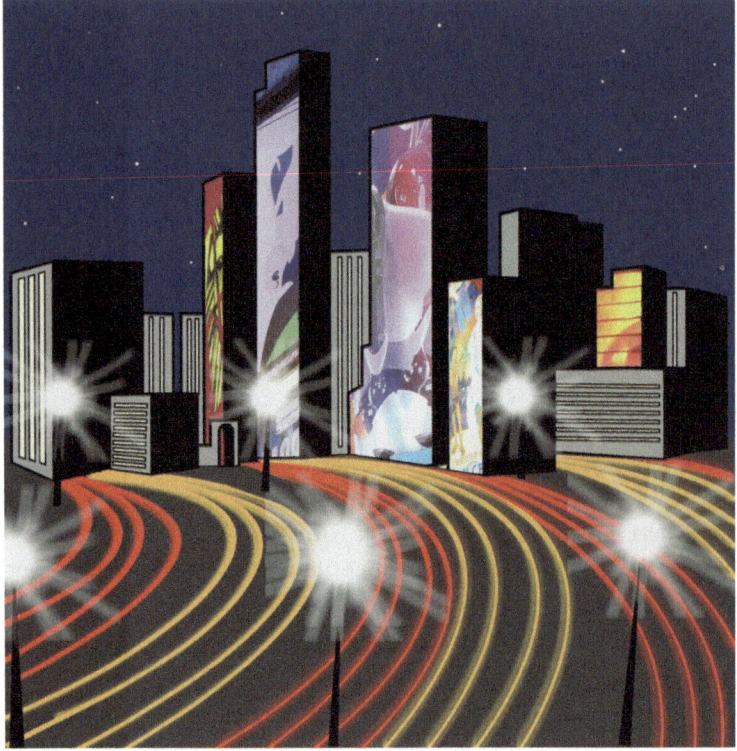

Figure 2.2 Neon city

a tube. The air is removed from the tube and the tube is subsequently filled with neon gas. When 15,000 volts of electricity are applied, the electrical discharge that occurs glows with a bright red-orange light. It can be turned blue with the addition of a small amount of mercury. Although still referred to as 'neon', all other colours are generated using the other noble gases or fluorescent lights of different colours. Neon is expensive but very small amounts are needed in lamps.

Neon is also used to make high-voltage indicators, lightning arrestors, wave meter tubes and TV tubes. Neon and helium are used in making gas lasers. Neon is also used as a coolant, for instance as a cryogenic refrigerant.

Reference

1   Royal Society of Chemistry. Available online at: http://www.rsc.org/periodic-table/element/10/neon

3

NEON MOTHER TINCTURE

The remedy was prepared in England by Jeremy Sherr at Helios Pharmacy in 1993. Analytical grade neon gas supplied by Fisons UK was bubbled through 14 ml of purified water for 10 minutes to make a 1:1000 solution (3×), (solubility 0.014 vol/vol).

The 2C was made by adding 0.4ml of 3× to 3.6ml of 50% ethanol B.P. and succussing the mixture. The 3C was made by adding one drop of the 2C solution to 99 drops (3.6ml) of 90% ethanol as per the Hahnemannian method. Higher potencies were made in a similar fashion.

For the proving 2g vials of sucrose pills were medicated with 2 drops of Neon 6C, 12C or 30C or with ethanol for placebo.

NEON 12C PHYSICAL AFFINITIES

The main affinities observed in the Neon proving were: Skin, head, eyes, iris, ears, nose, face, mouth, teeth, throat, abdomen, rectum, urinary, breasts and ovaries, upper and lower respiratory. For a complete list of physical symptoms please refer to the full proving.

Affinities observed clinically include: vertigo, headaches, influenza and colds, thyroid disorder, lack of appetite, anorexia, nausea, worms, **bladder**, abnormal menstrual bleeding and clots, uterine fibroids, speech and articulation, cough, carpal tunnel syndrome, perspiration, **itching**, warts, oedema, lack of coordination, numbness, twitching of muscles, pain in testes, crooked erections, ADD and HIV/AIDS. For full explanation of symptoms please see Chapter 12 Neon Cases.

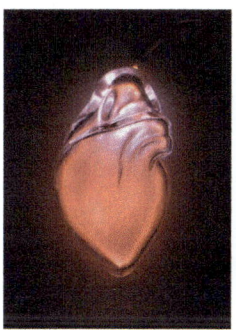 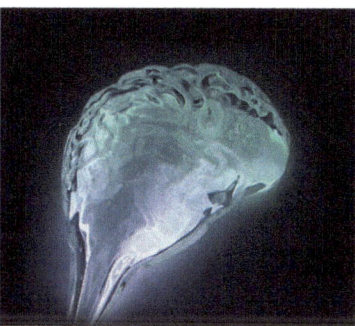 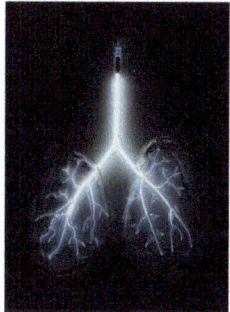

Figure 4.1 *Neon sculptures by Jessica Lloyd-Jones*

NEON 30C GENERALITIES

The following is a discussion of Neon's general symptoms.

Neon may experience a sensation of great strength and agility with easy and effortless walking. (Neon's neighbour Fluoric acid has a similar disposition for exercise). This highly energised state is opposed by a 'spaced out', drugged feeling, lack of energy, lethargy or a brittle sensation. Other features are awkwardness and clumsiness, sensations of extreme cold or heat and general dryness. The remedy has a morning and evening aggravation, especially at 6 p.m., as well as an aggravation on alternating days. A tendency to colds and 'flu' was observed, often with allergies, bloodshot, dry and tired eyes, lachrymation, sneezing, watery discharge, catarrh and inflammation of the throat. Provers experienced a variety of headaches, bad

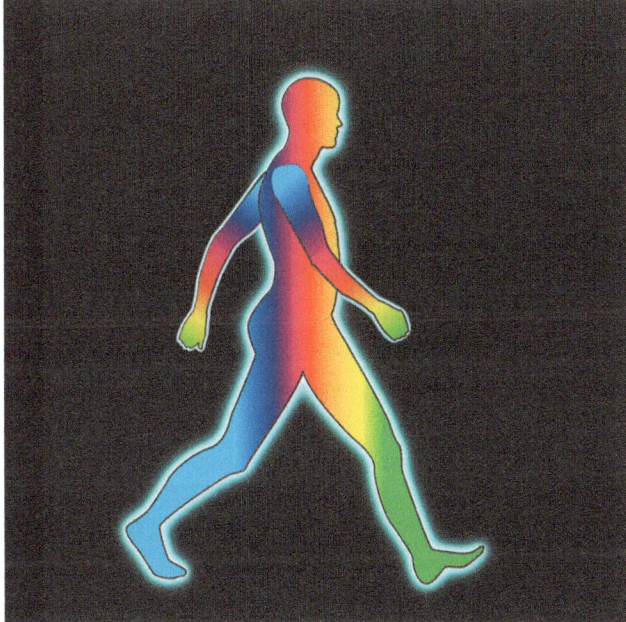

Figure 5.1 *Neon Man*

tastes in the mouth and toothaches. Neon may desire chocolate, green food, oranges, orange juice, refreshing things, ice or salt. Heartburn, nausea, flatulence and abdominal pains are among the more prominent digestive symptoms. There were cases of respiratory distress and pains in the back and extremities.

Neon is a psoric remedy. Itching and eruptions are prominent features. There is a general dryness, of mouth, skin, throat and stool and a desire for bathing, especially hot baths, but these may aggravate.

Neon has an affinity for colours. An unusual symptom is a disposition for glowing discharges and shiny, luminous discolourations of skin or in vision. Hearing and smell are acute with sensitivity to noise.

Neon relates to birth and the newborn, 'neo' meaning 'new'. Over-exposure to neon lights (for example, when babies are treated for jaundice) can be a causation of various ailments.

NEON 200C EMOTIONAL ESSENCE

Neon is rich in mental and emotional symptoms. Of course, not all of these symptoms need to be present in a Neon case, provided that the totality or essential meaning is similar to the remedy.

The Neon proving elicited many positive and enjoyable sensations and states. As one might expect in the proving of a noble gas, stillness and contentment were experienced along with a total lack of desire. Neon may be full of gratitude, an overwhelming appreciation for the world's beauty. This euphoric state was described as 'spaced out', 'joy', 'bliss', 'arriving home' or 'paradise'. There may be mental clarity, creativity and acute concentration. Some provers experienced a sensation of walking with effortless ease and with a sense of uprightness, freedom and agility. At best this elated state becomes a feeling of invincibility and oneness. Many of these sensations are characteristic of 'healthy noble gases'.

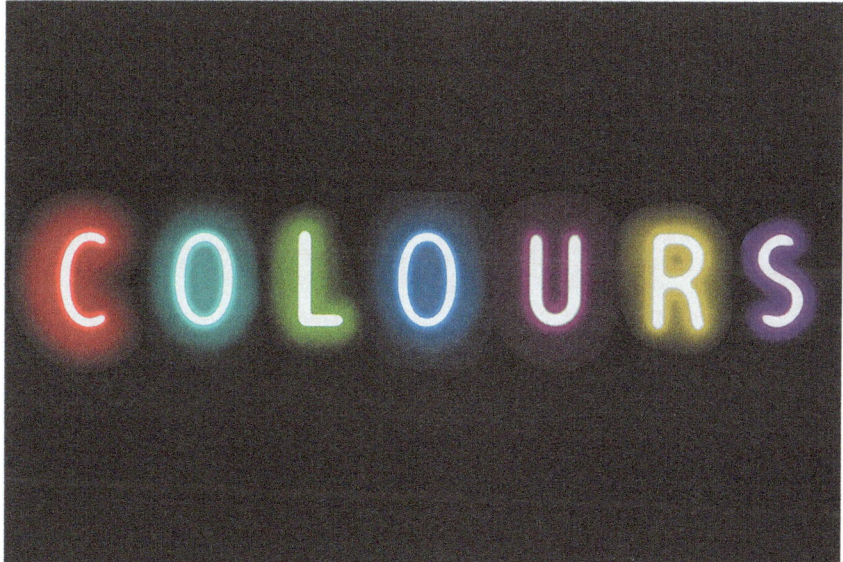

Figure 6.1 *Neon colours*

Just as we are drawn to the neon signs that illuminate our cities, Neon provers were attracted to lights and colours: clear blues, vivid greens, sparkling sapphires and jewels (Figure 6.1).

Neon has a strong affinity for water, which manifests in thoughts and dreams of oceans and rivers, of Noah's ark, the second day of creation and in sensations of dissolving or drowning. Neon is also fascinated by the sky and the stars. Provers experienced a feeling of being kissed by heaven and of harmony between heaven and earth. There is a yearning to reconnect with the stars, to reach beyond the sky to faraway stellar bodies. As the movie says, '*ET, go home!*'

A strange and recurring theme in the Neon proving was that of doors and windows. Provers would hear someone knocking at the door but on answering find that nobody was there. The intriguing opposite symptom was dreams of knocking on other people's doors. There may be a desire to spy on others, specifically through the keyhole.

In contrast to the feelings of unity and oneness, some provers experienced a sense of division. Another unusual characteristic was an attraction to numbers, especially even numbers, and an aversion to odd numbers.

Time is a recurrent theme in Neon, often involving a pleasant feeling of being present in the 'here and now'. On the other hand time may seem to rush forward into the future, often associated with speediness, rapid speech, impatience or clairvoyance. In extreme cases there may be a timeless confusion in which the thread connecting past to future is lost.

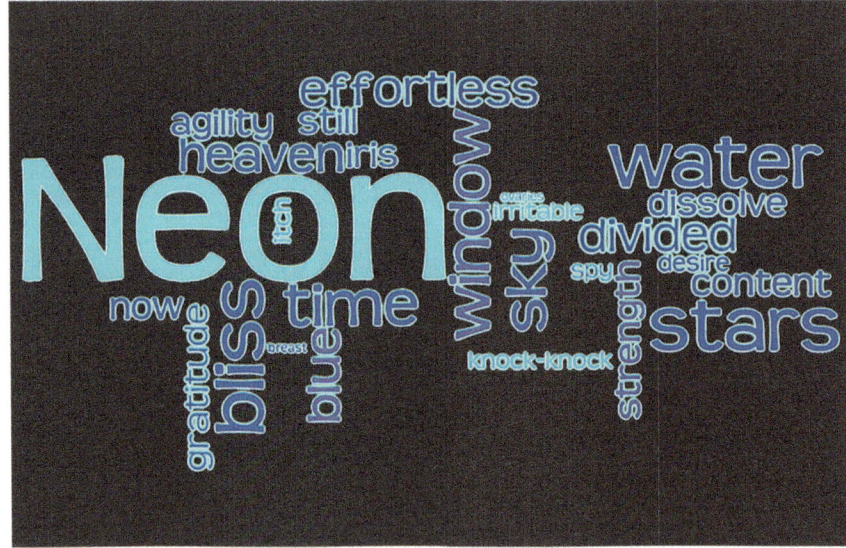

Figure 6.2 Neon wordle

There are several references in the proving to newborn babies, and indeed Neon may be childish or naïve. There is a need to be straightforward and to tell the truth, a symptom shared by some of the other noble gases.

NEON 1M HIGHER THEMES

There are two sides to every remedy. To understand the remedy fully we must perceive both sides and the nature of the split that separates the two. I mentioned in the introduction that while I had a good understanding of Neon's 'positive' side, I had neglected to study the opposite 'negative' side. Perhaps the attractive highlights had grabbed my attention. Floating on the surface of the Neon picture is an agile, blissful and contented state that outshines the less pleasant aspects, leaving them in the shadows. But while the positive side of a remedy may draw our attention, the negative side may be more important clinically. To elevate our perception to the next potency we will compare both sides of Neon, examining the nature of unification on the one hand and the results of division on the other.

Positive

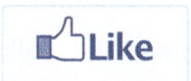

Contentment

At its best Neon produces a state of blissful contentment in the here and now, an enlightened and effortless ease of being. With a full complement of electrons in its outer shell, neon has no need to combine with any other element, manifesting a desireless state which is reflected in the following symptoms:

Sitting on the sofa, feeling very peaceful, there is a stillness inside me; it's all right to sit here and watch the world through my window. The absence of the urge to do anything strikes me.

Feel very calm and peaceful inside, no desire to busy myself with a hundred things.

I am contented – not operating so much through my emotions/feelings, which is unusual for me. It is as if there is a calm part of me underneath which I do not usually have access to because I am constantly being pulled this way and that way by thoughts and feelings popping into my head. Now my mind is free of these distractions and I feel contented.

Lost the compulsion for extravagant shopping; only bought what I needed.

Feeling comfortable, peaceful and contented.

I had a general feeling of not wanting anything, I felt totally un-needy.

Feel totally desireless. Nothing I need or want, a tremendous oneness. It feels like paradise.

Perhaps more than any other symptom, the following best illustrates the contented state of Neon: total fulfilment with a lack of any aspirations or desires.

This is like being given more than you ever wanted, like wanting the sun and being given the universe.

Tranquillity

Neon provers experienced a profound calmness. When one wishes for nothing there is no need to seek. Neon rests at its centre, motionless and tranquil. This is reminiscent of Helium, but is even more pronounced in Neon.

Feel calm and stable, with a greater awareness.

I am more relaxed, more in the present than usual. My mind is usually very busy and I do not just sit down and relax, but now I am less hurried and am able to sit down, gaze out of the window and listen to music. I would normally get tense about being late for an appointment, but now it does not bother me.

While cooking a meal for many people, usually a pressurised situation, I felt very happy and relaxed.

I have been less busy, meditating and reading, which I normally find hard to do.

Agility and effortless motion

Walking up a long gradual incline, I felt I was covering great distances with every stride. I felt I was doing the usual 20 minute walk in seconds. I felt like a titan in seven-league boots.

While walking in the fresh air, I suddenly felt as if I was cruising along on an energy which was not of my own muscular power. It seemed as if it was coming from somewhere else. It seemed effortless and unreal. I felt as if I was passing everyone else.

Walking is effortless, light and free. I have a sensation of walking uniformly. I feel so different in my body. I am all in the now, especially in my lower legs and feet. At last, I touch the earth.

Bliss

Ultimately Neon provers experienced a state of enlightened bliss. Everything happens in the here and now, and they feel at ease with the universe. If only our patients presented with such symptoms!

Today, walking around was like meditating – a sense of absolute oneness. It was like it was all happening and I was just observing. When I did Tai Chi, it felt effortless and blissful. I felt no resistance, a harmony between heaven and earth. I thought, 'It's great to be home.' I felt I had been travelling all my life (perhaps for many lifetimes) and now I was home.

I felt very steady, warm, peaceful, content, and blissful.

Singing out loud to myself. Ecstatic feeling. Everything seems more beautiful.

Moments of universal happiness.

Neon centres itself in the present moment.

Prior to taking the remedy, I felt too far in the future. I feel as if I have taken a step back and am in the here and now.

Usually I am distracted by thoughts coming into my mind but now I am more focused and less hurried.

These feelings result in a highly spiritual state.

Dream of being a successful spiritual teacher.

Dream of being in a crowd with a spiritual teacher.

It was as if there was no difference between the observer and the observed.

In my mind's eye I was in a desert. A wolf was looking kindly at me and asking 'why are you waiting?' It said, 'You're as resourceful and powerful a teacher as I am.' Second vision was of a small desert owl that said, 'You too can be wise and wonder with all-round vision.' An amazed wonder although also with a sense of wandering in the desert with the wolf.

The last symptom is reminiscent of Helium which also has all-round vision. If we combine the blissful feelings with the Neon affinity for water we get a sense of dissolving:

Had the strong thought, 'My connection with the past is dissolving'.

Dreamt that I was 'Aquarius'. I was pleased about it though I had no idea what this meant.

Alongside this bliss are forgiveness and a total absence of guilt as identity melts into the One.

I now feel forgiven for the ultimate sin. I feel unbounded love for myself but I wonder, 'Is there a "me" anymore?' No more separations!!

Somehow I had a very profound realisation that this is my own life time. My usual feelings of guilt shifted and I was able to take responsibility for my own life.

I feel totally clean inside and out. I have lost the unclean feeling I always had.

The bliss and melting of boundaries result in a profound state of gratitude.

Woke extremely happy with feelings of gratitude.

Heart is full to overflowing with no boundaries. Tears of joy and gratitude. Great pleasure from and desire for far horizons.

We may summarise all the above in one short sentence:

Dissolving of boundaries as the ego melts into the whole, here and now.

I felt bathed in warmth and light. I lost the isolation of myself being myself. It was the most gentle feeling I had ever had in my life. My centre was immovable with great stillness. No thoughts flitted around – just awareness. There are no words to describe it. What I thought of as the normal 'me' was actually everywhere. There was no separation. There wasn't a 'me', my identity was still there but with no boundaries. This is like being given more than you ever wanted, like wanting the sun and being given the universe. Before, I just wanted enlightenment, but now I am aware that there are higher states of consciousness. I have set my sights higher.

A truly noble state!

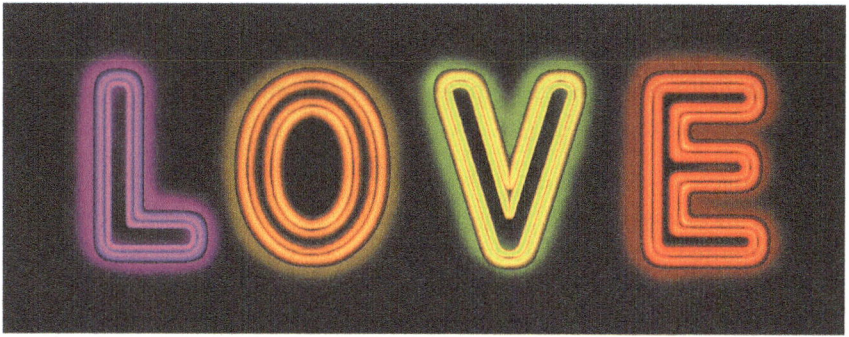

Figure 7.1 Love

Negative

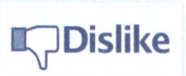

I am a star in the firmament
that observe the world, despises the world
and consumed in its heat.

Hermann Hesse[1]

While the positive symptoms seem highly desirable they may not be as clinically useful as the negative aspects. I will now delve into the negative side, for therein lies the pathology in the majority of cases. For this exploration I will use three approaches:

1. Application of the law of opposites to speculate on the nature of the negative side of the remedy.
2. A re-examination of the proving itself.
3. A mini-meditation proving.

Using opposites to speculate on the nature of the negative side

Every remedy has two opposite actions, sometimes referred to as primary and secondary. When a remedy seems one-sided we can speculate on its opposite side. However, in many cases an opposite cannot be accurately determined. What is the opposite of a tomato? A cucumber? Or perhaps a lemon? What is the opposite of an ulcer? In some cases a precise opposite does not exist while in others there may be an array of possibilities. Nevertheless, because each facet of the remedy is covered by numerous, clearly described symptoms, we can use the totality to predict the opposite side. I have listed below some key features of Neon together with possible opposites. We will later examine if these are corroborated by the proving or by clinical experience.

- Connected – Separated
- One – Divided
- Contented – Discontent, dissatisfaction
- Perfect – Imperfect
- Freedom from desire – Bound by desire; addiction
- Stillness – Restlessness
- In the present – Holding on to the past or rushing towards the future
- Tranquillity – Anxiety, irritability
- Awareness – Lack of awareness, locked in self
- Gratitude – Selfish ingratitude
- Bliss – Wretchedness
- No original sin – Continuous sin
- Spiritual – Materialistic
- Freedom from identity and the past – Enslaved by identity and history
- Letting go – Holding on
- Dissolving of boundaries – Bound; imprisoned
- Elation – Drugs
- Water – Earth
- Stars– Our planet
- Even – Odd
- Paradise – Hell

Hence there is a possibility that Neon, at its worst, would be discontent, dissatisfied, full of desires, restless, dwelling on the past, rushing towards the future, anxious, irritable, locked in self, separated, divided, selfish, ungrateful, wretched, sinful, materialistic, enslaved by identity, history and addictions, earth-bound or the odd man out. A living hell!

We should also keep in mind that many of the positive effects of the proving were curative. If we focus on the symptoms that disappeared during the proving (marked in the next two symptoms in bold) we find that Neon can have an addictive personality with a tendency to work-aholism and compulsive consumerism.

Feel very calm and peaceful inside, no desire to **busy myself with a hundred things**.

Lost the compulsion for **extravagant shopping**; only bought what I needed.

Feel out of control, as if time is moving relentlessly and remorselessly forward and I'm stuck behind, unable to keep up. Panic, guilt, constant anxiety that I won't get it all done.

Added to this is a state of selfishness. Neon, driven by its desires, is attracted by the bright city lights, which promise gratification but deliver addiction:

During the proving there has been a shift of focus to my own needs.

Thus instead of:

This is like being given more than you ever wanted, like wanting the sun and being given the universe.

I would synthesise the discontent state of Neon as:

This is like constant unfulfilled desire, like being promised the sun and being given a yellow neon light.

These are the possibilities. Let us proceed to the provings.

'Negative' aspects of the proving

The speculations of the previous section bear out well in the proving. Neon produced quite a number of unpleasant emotions including confusion, indifference, loneliness, estrangement, depression, grief, self-disgust, wretchedness, discontent, guilt, anxiety, hurriedness, stress, irritability, reproach of self and of others, anger, cursing and violence.

To illustrate these emotions more clearly, I have edited, combined and abbreviated several provers into an 'As If One Person' (AIOP) monologue. It would be instructive to read it in one go in order to internalise the Neon 'state'.

Wound up confused and out of my centre. Can't generate any excitement. Indifference towards the dirty house. I leave the dishes and dirty hair in the bath. I can't be bothered to write my book; I don't want to do this anymore. I am withdrawn and grouchy, want to be alone. Staying in bed a lot. Detached, withdrawn from emotions. Feeling: 'I am there for everyone but no one is ever there for me.' I feel alone, as if everyone perceives me as odd. I feel strange, like an outsider, and I cannot connect on any level. Very subdued and depressed. It feels like a void. No joy in the birds singing. 'How can I lift it?' Great sadness and hopelessness; I cried and cried. Weeping on waking. Low in the morning. Desperate. Want to cry all the time. I'm in the 'Valley of Discontent'. Burst into tears. Sad and depressed. Listless, low energy. Want to close my eyes. I don't feel like working and just want to go to sleep or read under the covers. I thought about my grandfather and cried over his unfortunate life. Fed-up because things are not as they should be. I feel disgusted with myself; violent and malicious. God, I feel so wretched. Out of control, as if time is moving relentlessly and remorselessly forward and I am stuck behind. Panic, guilt, constant anxiety that I won't get it all done. Anxious about everything and depressed about the anxiety, it feels all wrong. More stress than usual – feels like an ordeal. Great irritability from noise and from being spoken to. Had an explosion about not being the perfect person. Irritable after a dream. Irritable, argumentative and sharp. I became very aggressive and blew a fuse at one of our visitors. I reproach my partner. Cursing and swearing. Irritable in the afternoon, smouldering away in the kitchen, like an explosion. Get up late in a horrible mood and reproach my partner again. I hurt him but I don't care. Indifferent, malicious and vindictive, full of hatred. I want to reproach people. I've been in a rotten mood all day, dwelling on past offenses. I just can't let go, it's making me angry. 'I'll kill you', 'I'll slit your throat.' Violent, irritable and aggressive. I am really pissed off at the situation. I feel out of control and helpless and lash out with vehemence and anger at the situation and myself.

At its lowest point the negative feelings of Neon combine with its 'watery oblivion' to generate a sensation of drowning in woes, a sharp contrast to the gentle dissolving of the ego.

I woke up with the feeling that **I was drowning**. I could not catch my breath. I reached out for my wife to help me. It was quite disturbing **not being able to catch my breath. An emotional wave** came over me and I wanted to sob.

To sum up: Neon may feel depressed, discontented, anxious, guilty or stressed. Feelings of irritability and anxiety may develop into anger, reproachfulness, cursing or violent thoughts. The calm stillness can deteriorate into an 'inert' or apathetic depression characterised by indifference, alternating moods, sadness or dwelling, a dissatisfied state described as a 'wretched feeling' or the 'Valley of Discontent'. In contrast to the gratitude, there may be a feeling of not being appreciated, 'I am here for everyone yet no one is here for me'. Some provers experienced disorientation, a sense of being out of their centre. Others felt like aliens or strangers, with an inability to recognise people or objects. Like odd numbers, Neon provers were the odd ones out.

Many of these unpleasant symptoms are common to a number of remedies. Neon patients may easily be confused with the common essences of Nux vomica, Natrum muriaticum, Aurum, Kali phosphoricum and many other depressed, irritable and explosive remedies. Ideally, therefore, we would need to see both sides of the remedy in one patient in order to make an accurate prescription. For instance:

Depressed, but there are moments of universal happiness and love that flicker in amidst the depressed state.

Drugs

Some of the emotional states seen in the proving, especially the 'spaced out' feelings, suggest that Neon could be a remedy for drug addiction. The descriptions seem to indicate acute, drug-like experiences. It remains to be seen whether the remedy could be suitable for the chronic tendencies underlying drug addictions. I have no clinical experience with this aspect of Neon, and can only assume the possibility from the negative aspects and the mini-meditation proving. The following are Neon symptoms which relate to acute drug states, combined into an 'As if one person' (AIOP) description:

It's reminiscent of taking hallucinogens. Buzzy, cut-off feeling. Feeling spaced out. Recognise a change in awareness – a vaguely stoned, unreal feeling. Giggly, childish, grinning. Feel light, as if I'm coming down from drugs; very spacey and light – headed. Super relaxed, can't read, can't concentrate. I feel spacey and happier than usual. I don't quite seem to know where my body is in space, tripping and falling. Shortly after taking the remedy, I was confused about where I was. Feel not connected, not in control, as if in a dream. Intoxicated feeling. Light-headed, a sense of speediness and hurry. Exhausted, drained, woolly feeling.

The whole dream was in dark colours – depressing and bleak. All except the classroom scene, which was warm and light. Yet that was when I felt angry and tricked. It was all too brave-new-world cheerful and involved deceit.

Meditation proving

The following is a 'Mini Meditation' (MM) proving. Please skip this section if you feel uncomfortable with such provings. I have done my share of full Hahnemannian provings and will continue to do them. But alongside the classical provings I have experimented with meditation provings, in which the prover holds the remedy in their hand or sleeps with it under their pillow or uses similar means of proximity and induction. There are certain advantages to a mini meditation proving, provided that it is conducted with a highly sensitive person: it is quick and often provides an unusual perspective. It is *essential* that the prover be blind to the remedy.

It is important to understand that such a proving can only offer suggestions for materia medica as an adjunct to full provings. The test is whether the symptoms match the totality and essence of the conventional proving, and whether they are borne out in clinic. Many of the meditation provings I have conducted alongside classical ones have proved their validity in clinic.

My wife Camilla, having participated in 17 Hahnemannian provings and having edited several more, has developed the sensitivity and acuity of senses to produce excellent mini meditation provings. She is quite clairvoyant, being born to a line of psychically sensitive people. Her MM provings are unexpected, vivid and highly accurate. I particularly appreciate that, in contrast to many of the 'nicer' provings, she often reveals the 'negative' side of a remedy.

In the Neon MM proving Camilla had no idea what the remedy was. We both held a very different image of Neon, one of bliss, water and numbers, which contrasted sharply with the symptoms she experienced, and she was extremely surprised when she found out what the remedy was. Her proving was a revelation to us, but it made sense, and has since proved very useful in clinic.

The proving was recorded verbatim from the moment it began.

MM proving of Neon

Laughing: I'd better get a Nobel Prize for this, haha (or maybe YOU should get a Nobel Prize for this).

Itchy and restless (she is scratching). Itchy gums and tingling behind my teeth. The itching is changing places.

Restless and irritable. Restless legs.

Sighing.

Teeth clenched.

Feels like everything is on the surface! Irritated with the itch. This is not really real, it's very much on the surface. It feels skin-deep, on the skin only. Itching here and there – legs, head, wandering itch, annoying, irritating.

Hard to grasp this one (this proving).

Feels like a young man who wants to play football.

I feel out of it! Light-headed and out of it. I feel drugged. Like a high vibe or sound, like 'eeeeeeeeee', not pleasant. I feel like an irritable, highly revved drug addict, a junkie. I feel like a junkie – skinny, restless, itching. I need a fix.

This remedy is all about nerves. Nerves on the surface. Skin-deep, not much more, skin-deep mentally and physically. Nothing deep going on, just itching and the desire for a fix.

It feels like my existence is reduced to the moment of getting my fix, the drugs, nothing else matters, so skin-deep. I don't know what's underneath. This is just a cover. I feel like an adolescent boy. I don't feel like me.

I want to just go into oblivion, don't know if it's a death wish. Desire not to be.

Adolescent boy, drug addict, itch and scratch and fix, brainless, just a desire that has to be fulfilled, that's all there is to it, drugs or theft. Like an itch that has to be scratched, nothing more, you can't help it.

An addict! A 17- or 18-year-old adolescent, I think.

This is an add-on layer, the end result. It could have been any story before the addiction.

This is true addiction, not just an extra glass of wine.

You have an itch and you just have to scratch, so your life becomes smaller and smaller: no depth, no history, no future. All that matters is where you can get your next fix, that's it. Nothing complex about it.

'Ask me my favourite colour!' (*JS: this is a shared joke of ours about a young self-centred teenager we know.*) Haha: black is my favourite colour, and studs and leather.

Young and dumb: you try something (a drug) and it takes over, you lose your dreams, goals and desires, you lose who you are. All you have left is an itch that needs to be scratched. So, like junkies you must detox first so that the itching and scratching stop, then you can start digging deeper. You cannot avoid the scratching, it's too strong and it takes over your life, loves and values. You are reduced to itching and scratching. You have to deal with that first on the surface. I don't know who is underneath this, it could be anyone. It could be the result of an accident.

No emotions, this person doesn't care. Totally indifferent to everything. Life is reduced to the here and now, but not a healthy one, a false here and now.

This is like a miasm because it comes from the outside, not from within. Not like a real disease but like an add-on, like someone says, 'from now on you wear a red hat'. It is so strong, a stronger dissimilar disease, you cannot fight it. The itch is so powerful, you must scratch, then you become a reduced form of yourself. The inner who is gone, the hat takes over.

JS: What would the opposite side be?

Someone who single-mindedly pursues something, someone addicted to a career, a job or a goal, someone with a really strong passion for their work, to the point that they can't see any other life beyond. All else becomes insignificant, loved ones, holidays, the mundane things of life. The project or mission completely takes over and consumes the person without their realising it.

Like a kind of selfishness, it's all about me, me, me. Me, myself and I. Living in my own bubble.

JS: What would the healthy image of the remedy be?

Someone between the junkie and the alpha male workaholic, but in a positive way. Someone with drive and vision but also an awareness of others, an understanding of the 'bigger picture' and the knowledge that there is more to life than work

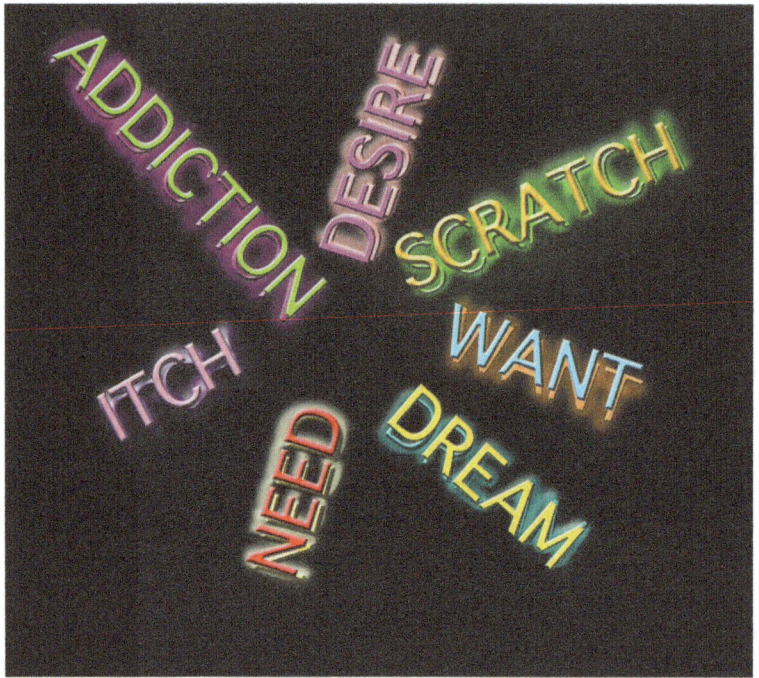

Figure 7.2 *'The Itchy Scratchy Show'*

Comment

This proving represents the extreme negative side of Neon as exemplified by the previous sections. We see a simplistic, two-dimensional personality, everything is on the surface. With the first shot of heroin, the soon-to-be junkie experiences extreme bliss and contentment. The secondary reaction soon follows – desperate need and slavery to an addiction. The desireless state is replaced by a condition dominated purely by desire, the result of a randomly acquired severe addiction. Enlightenment and the melting of ego give way to a skin-deep and selfish superficiality. The stars are replaced by the false glow of city neon and man is reduced to a child-like state of dependency.

This reminds me of a quote from Kent.[2]

In one all to hate, and in the other all to love.
In the one despised, in the other beloved.
The one, then, is man with his love for the degrees of uses; the other but an image with his hatred of uses.
In man is heaven; in his image is hell.
The fullness of man is but his capacity for growth as a receptacle for love, wisdom and use.
The image of man is hatred, ignorance, and to be cared for by local protectors and penitentiaries.
Independence contrasted with dependence.
Freedom contrasted with bondage.
Inconceivable gradations exist between these extremes. These varying shades of changes in man come by inheritance, vocation, opportunity, disease and drugs.

Conclusion

The three tools which I have used to elucidate the negative picture: opposites, the proving itself and the meditation proving, echo each other and fit together to create a comprehensive whole. Naturally, the clinical picture does not have to be as intense. The main theme, however, should be there:

We are attracted by the neon lights of the city that promise the sun in the dark of night, but deliver a superficial empty experience, the Valley of Discontent.

There is no greater sin than desire,
No greater curse than discontent,
No greater misfortune than wanting something for oneself.
Therefore he who knows that enough is enough will always have enough.

Tao Te Ching[3]

References

1   Hermann Hesse: *Quotes*. Available online at: http://www.goodreads.com/quotes/234534-i-am-a-star-in-the-firmament-that-observe-the

2   Kent JT. 'The Trend of Thought Necessary for the Comprehension and Retention of the Application of the Homoeopathic Materia Medica'. in *New Remedies, Clinical Cases, Lesser Writings, Aphorisms and Precepts*. New Delhi: B. Jain Publishers Pvt. Ltd, 1998. p. 461.

3   LaoTzu. *Tao Te Ching* (trans. Feng G, English J). New York NY: Vintage Books, 1972. Chapter 46.

8

NEON 10M SPIRITUAL THEMES

One divided

To potentise our understanding of Neon to the 10M level, we will investigate the proving fractals as multiple manifestations of a single idea.[i] The first theme to emerge is a sense of union, of becoming one, represented by the 'As if one person' amalgamation below:

I saw two points of white light merging together, becoming one. A sense of absolute oneness. It was as if there was no difference between the observer and the observed. I lost the isolation of myself being myself. I feel like an unfertilised egg, no division.

The opposite of this oneness is a sensation of division, reflected in the following symptoms:

Felt I could divide. Image of being split down the middle (left and right sides split).

Sensation of division in my head: left side clear, light and cool, right side warm, muzzy and dense.

Sensation that the top of my head was rising while I and the rest of my body were sinking, like a horizontal separation.

I have been living without a partner for 10 years, which I have really enjoyed. Now I have the uncomfortable feeling of needing a partner. This is a feeling of only being half and needing another.

---

[i] A fractal is a mathematical concept of repeated, self-similar patterns.

As if one person

One person,
as if
Fragmented by the winds of life
and ravaged by desire,
disintegrated
body soul
faltering to trial
antagonising will and
mind your inner liar
the coolness of your brain
extinguishing your fire
while restless legs
are running nights
and joints are turning stiff
Then unaware
you come to me,
as if one being,
As if.

Numbers

Pure mathematics is, in its way, the poetry of logical ideas.

Albert Einstein[1]

I just read last year 4,153,237 people got married. I don't want to start any trouble, but shouldn't that be an even number?

Bill Murray (Twitter)[2]

It is apparent that one of the essential ideas of Neon is the polarity of oneness opposing division. The first whole number that can be divided is two, and Neon abounds with twos and its multiples. The affinity for numbers may indicate a predilection for mathematics, but the main idea is the number two itself. Neon completes the second period, which may explain its attraction to even numbers.

I've always really liked odd numbers. I suddenly feel the capacity to be even. Even numbers are much more attractive. I feel like I've never known even numbers and now I do. Half was missing. It is like a new toy of evenness.

Occasional thoughts about numbers: I have always felt comfortable with odd numbers. Now, being both gives a whole other dimension. To have had half missing for so long! What is different? From 3 to 1: slight tension. From 2 to 1: effortless, natural progression.

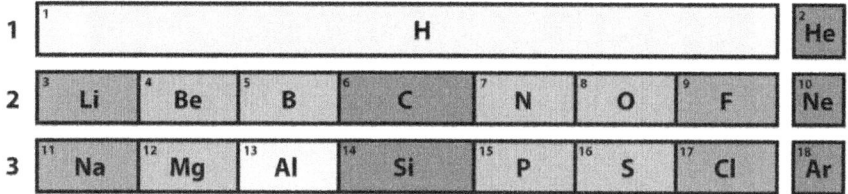

Figure 8.1 *The second period bridging the first and third periods*

Thoughts about odd and even numbers. I had always jumped down from 3 to 1. That made me too high. I now feel that I need to work my way down, 3-2-1. In the past, it was easier for me to go up than to come down. Now I feel that I can go either way.

These symptoms suggest that the progression between numbers is as important as the numbers themselves. We can relate this to the evolution of the periodic table. Neon is the bridge between the first and third periods, as illustrated in Figure 8.1 and by the following symptom:

I had the sensation of being between two different experiences.

The preceding period containing Hydrogen and Helium is characterised by oneness, the journey from the homogeneous, collective universal soul to the single, individual soul. Neon represents the first division. We will see that the whole of the second period is occupied with the process of division, a process which is completed in Neon.

Illustrations of the neon atom display an extraordinary degree of even symmetry. Given that neon is element number 10 and that its atom contains 10 protons and 10 electrons, it is not surprising to find the number 20 featuring in the proving. Here are a few examples:

Dreamt of a huge construction whose centre was covered by a tarpaulin with 20 spokes radiating from it. A man beside me counted and said there were 20. I thought, 'Good, that's 2 × 10.'

Dream . . . she said the mirror belonged to somebody in Room 20. I searched upstairs and downstairs for room 20. . . .

Though Helium represents one, deep within its roots we can perceive the susceptibility to Neon's division.

It feels like I am stepping from the oneness to the twoness. (Helium)

Out of the darkness light was born. . . . Connecting us to life. One two, one two. (Helium)

I felt only half here, yet I was functioning very well. I felt clear, efficient, light and calm, as if I had left my other half in a dream. Each half felt

Figure 8.2 *Neon separation of yin and yang*

complete. Each half was very complete as though whole but it was half. (Helium)

> The Tao begot one
> The one begot two . . .
> Two begot choice

> Adapted from the *Tao Te Ching*[3]

When Neon splits into two, Yin and Yang split (Figure. 8.2), separating from each other and generating future and past, forwards and backwards, desires and aversions and ultimately, choice.

Choice

> The all-encompassing, nameless, holy, whole begot One. (He let it go)
> Now felt quite important.
> Here was also justifiably proud.
> Somehow One thought he had created himself. (Oops!)
> But there was No-one to appreciate that.
> One had had enough!
> She decided to split.
> Just then Paradox arrived.
> After faced Before as Future took a step back.
> And Choice laughed.

Ova, pregnancy and birth

The idea of unity is further represented in Neon by a single ovum before fertilisation, and consequent cell division, takes place.

I felt like I was an unfertilised egg, an ovum, very peaceful.
Felt like thousands of ova sitting there waiting, with the thought that they were all female, complete and unfertilised.

By the process of splitting, unity begets diversity. Neon means new, and new things are born from division.

There is a new order in space.
Feeling increasing new life with every breath.

Neon represents the final stage of meiosis, the division of reproductive cells into gametes. These gametes, sperm and ova, unite into one zygote, a single cell from which two new cells are born and pregnancy begins. AIOP:

Dreamt I was pregnant. Dreams of pregnancy and labour. Dreamt that my sister and I had a house where old people could have babies. Dreamt I was in labour, lying with another pregnant woman in a warm bath.

Symbolically pregnancy spans from Helium to Neon. Helium relates to the incarnation of the soul, symbolising conception and the first month of pregnancy. The eight elements of the second period represent the following eight months of pregnancy. In this model, Lithium represents the second month, Beryllium the third and so on, culminating in a Neon delivery.

I had the sensation of being in transition in labour – the space between the dilation phase and the pushing phase. It felt like a big letting go.
Images of newborn babies crying.
On receiving photos of my newborn niece, I had tears of joy.
Dream of babies and their umbilical cords.

There are several parallels between the Neon picture and labour. When the foetus is enclosed in the uterine capsule, surrounded by the waters of birth, it longs to burst its shell and transit into a new world. Neon may prove to be a good remedy in labour or 'never been well since' delivery, as illustrated by some of the cases that I have included in Chapter 12.

The second day

And God said: 'Let there be a firmament in the midst of the waters, and let it divide the waters from the waters.' And God made the firmament, and divided the waters which were under the firmament from the waters which were above the firmament; and it was so. And God called the firmament Heaven. And there was evening and there was morning, a second day.

Genesis 1:6–8[4]

In the story of the seven days of creation Helium is analogous to the first day and Neon to the second. On the first day God separates light and darkness. On the second day the heavenly waters above are separated from the earthly waters below.

I had many thoughts about the second day of creation.

I have always felt comfortable with the division between the dark and the light. What I now need is the division between the heavens and the oceans. Thoughts about my love for the Pacific Ocean.

The upper and lower waters are separated by a firmament, which literally means the vault of heaven, sky. A support, prop, stay, equivalent to firma: to strengthen, support.

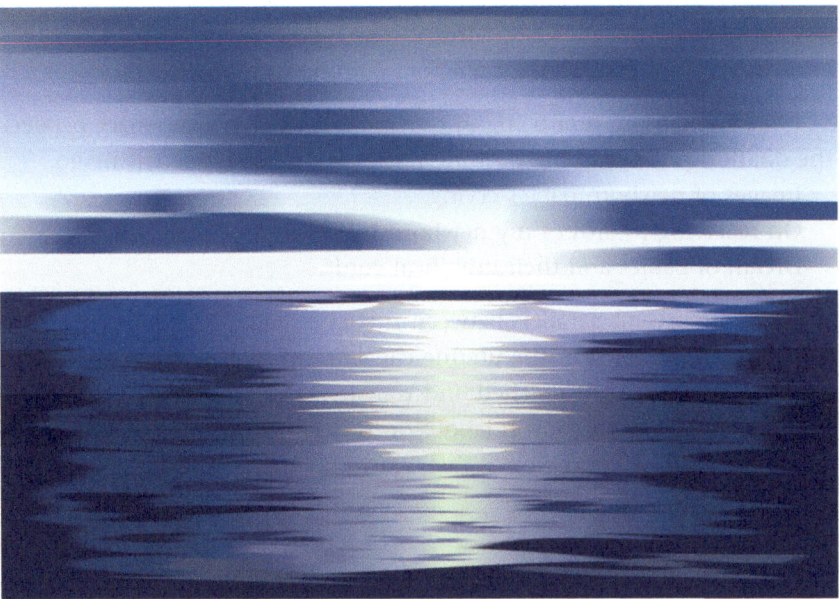

Figure 8.3 Waters above and below separate

The second day tells the story of vertical division. The waters above become the sky, and the waters below become the seas (Figure 8.3). In the human body the higher waters are tears, saliva, brain and spinal fluid, while the earth waters – urine and uterine fluids – lie below the diaphragm.

Water is created towards the end of the second period. Two hydrogen atoms combine with an atom of oxygen, element number eight, to form H_2O: 10 protons and 10 electrons. Neon mimics the water molecule by also holding 10 protons and 10 electrons. Now we are fluid.

Thoughts and dreams of rivers and oceans and being very happy near them.

I have superbly fluid and graceful motions, as if I were moving in water instead of air.

A phrase from a Lewis Carroll poem (see page 54) repeated itself over and over in my mind:

I saw an aged, aged man,
A-sitting on a gate.
"Who are you, aged man?" I said,
"And how is it you live?"
And his answer trickled through my head,
Like water through a sieve.

I felt this was about dissolving, which related to my feeling during the proving.

I have lost the delusion, which I have always had, that I could walk on water.

The analogy of the second day repeats in the story of Noah's ark. The whole world is submerged in flood waters and the animals board the ark two by two: water and division. The world survives through Noah's upright-ness, a righteous man.

Thoughts of twos and water. Saw images of Noah's ark.

I had thoughts of albatrosses circumnavigating the earth without having to touch the ground.

Dreamt that it rained all night and that I couldn't get my head above the water. The water levels were too high.

The second day of creation is characterised by the formation of a firma-ment. But what is this firmament and how does it manifest in our own world and in the world about us? In the following sections I will describe several analogies of the firmament as derived from the proving, namely stars, doors, windows, eyes, intellect and skin.

Firmament

Stars

> Man is a microcosm, or a little world, because he is an extract from all the stars and planets of the whole firmament, from the earth and the elements; and so he is their quintessence.
>
> Paracelsus[5]

The firmament separates us from the heavens above. Perhaps it is symbolised by the ozone layer which colours the twilight skies in a bluish-black hue (Figures 8.3, 8.4 and 8.5). Neon experiences a craving to return to the stars, to penetrate the firmament. It is interesting to remember that neon originates when carbon is burned in high-mass stars and is ejected into the galaxy by supernovae.

I just long for some clear nights so I can see my stars. If I could reconnect, then everything would be all right.

While lying awake in bed last night I heard a dinging sound, like glass or the sound of icicles tapping against each other. I looked but couldn't locate it. I tried to ignore it but the sound increased. I got up, went to the bedroom window and looked out over the back garden. It was a fantastic, cold, clear night. With a thrill of excitement I watched all the stars in the sky above and I just knew that the noise I'd heard was the stars trying to

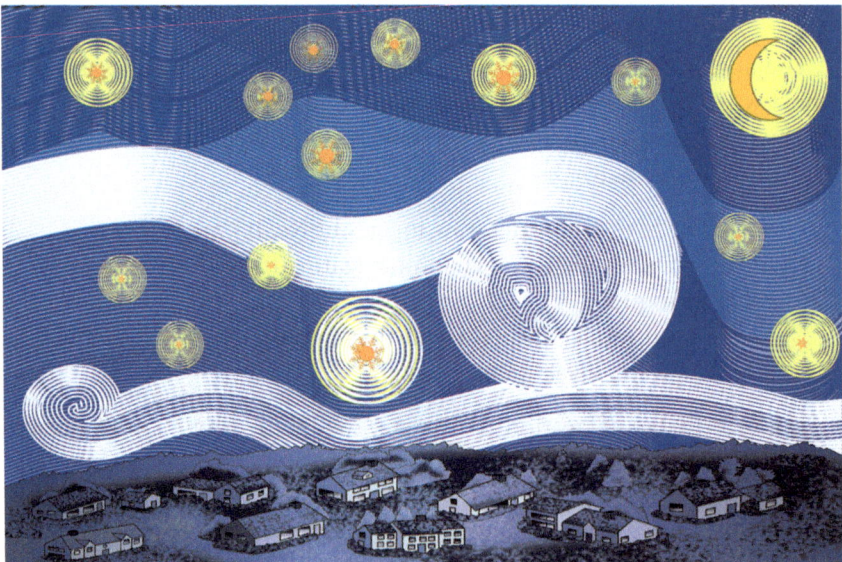

Figure 8.4 *Starry night*

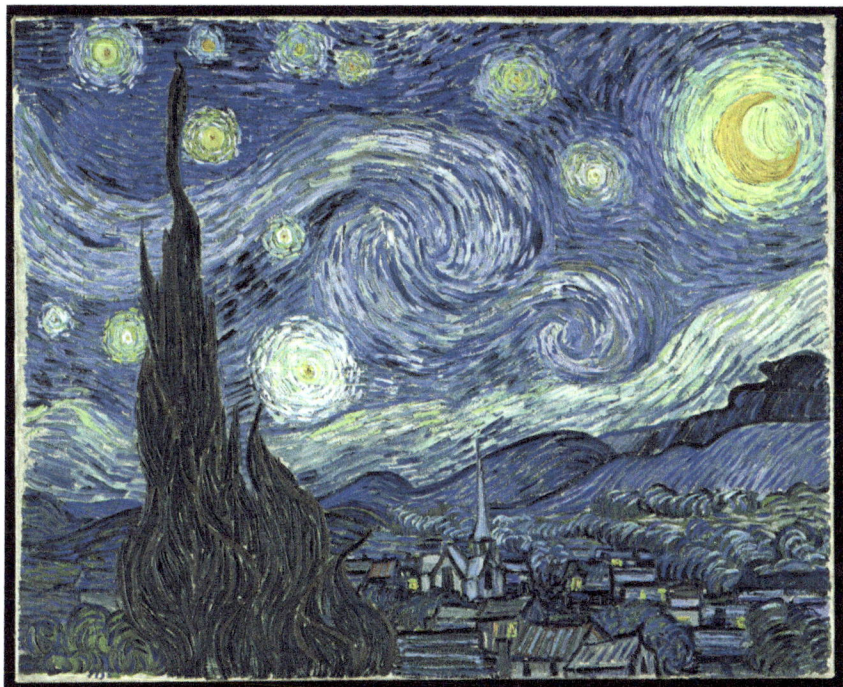

Figure 8.5 Starry night, Van Gogh

communicate with me. The noise seemed to last for ages. The thrill lasted for as long as I stood by the window. When I went back to bed I felt wonderful. The noise stopped.

Looking out of the window at the night sky, it suddenly cracked open and a great darkness revealed itself. Infinity was blackness. It was deeply disturbing.

Felt wonderful. Kept going outside during the night between midnight and 3 a.m. At last the sky was clear, moon brilliant, stars familiar, air cold. I felt so much a part of everything again.

While looking at a star map it looked unfamiliar, as if I had always been seeing the stars from the other side.

Dreamt I was studying a map of a 'space route' leaving from Australia, going to the moon, then to Jupiter and beyond.

I didn't feel I was on the planet at all.

This firmament or barrier sometimes appears as clouds. On a cloudy day I really wanted blue.

Vision was a little cloudy, like looking through a thin veil or light fog.

Clouds, clouds, where is the sky?

Doors and windows

Neon longs to return to the source, to feel the heavens and the stars, to perceive clear truth, to re-experience the watery comfort of our mother's uterus. But the division, the barrier, is always there. I felt this acutely during the proving, a sensation that my cosmic egg was longing to crack so that I could reunite with a higher truth. In other provers this was symbolised by the strange recurring phenomenon of people knocking on the door.

Twice thought I heard someone at the door, but when I checked there was no one there.

Twice I was awakened by the sound of a doorbell. I leapt out of bed to open the door, but no one was there.

Dreamt that I was knocking on many different doors. Nobody opened them.

A number of patients were knocking on the door and phoning me up to tell me they were well and to thank me.

'*Knock, knock, Neo*' from the film *The Matrix*.[6]

A similar idea was represented by windows. These windows may be portals to a beautiful world, or they may be occluded or derelict.

Dreams of windows.

Dream of a beautiful view over the sea from the balcony window.

Dreamt of being somewhere incredibly beautiful, looking out of the window and wanting to be out to enjoy it.

There is a stillness inside me; it's all right to sit here and watch the world through my window.

I sit down, gaze out of the window and listen to music.

The thrill lasted as long as I stood by the window.

Looking out of the window at the night sky.

I dreamt about a derelict building and derelict windows.

Dream of being locked out and climbing in through a small window.

I dreamt I was in my house but it was different and much older. A lot of the windows were in very bad condition. Suddenly one of the windows in front of the house fell out into the street and injured someone.

Another manifestation of our yearning to penetrate this 'firmament' is the desire to spy on others through the keyhole.

I notice a foolish and irresistible desire to spy on my partner through the keyhole of the door to his study. I now remember doing this a couple of times yesterday (the first day of the proving). I am finding it ridiculous, laughing to myself. I feel like a mischievous child, doing something he shouldn't do, giggling away to myself. It makes me feel excited in a childish sense. I have never felt compelled to spy on anyone ever – be it through a keyhole or otherwise.

My partner is having a bath. I resist the urge to go and watch him through the keyhole of the bathroom door. However, a strong desire to go up and spy on him lingers in my mind.

Neon, a soul manifested in an embryo, is at the stage of venturing into a new world. It does not know what is waiting there, but is ready to take the first step once the door opens. A state of stillness and bliss lies within, but this bliss is tainted with expectation. Once Neon steps through the door, a new world of temptation awaits, a world full of division, desire and sin.

Sensation of waiting.

A friend said, 'I have never seen you look so well. You look like you are waiting for something – a bolt out of the blue.'

Window of the soul

Another representation of the firmament is the iris, the barrier of our eye, through whose window, the pupil, we can see. Our eyes both perceive and separate us from reality, forming a window between the outside world and our distorted perception of it.

Image of being inside my iris and looking through it. I saw a large iris and I was looking through it. From the centre of it light was radiating out.

With eyes closed, I felt the right eye was seeing light through the iris of an eye in front of me.

In the proving of Helium I mentioned that when the soul enters the body it splits in two, one half migrating forward towards the iris and the other retreating to the shadows. This process is completed in Neon, as the identity settles in the iris. Henceforth we believe what we see and deny that which is hidden in the gloomy recesses of our subconscious. We believe that we reside in our eyes. It is said that the eyes are the window of the soul. Our mistake is that we imagine our eyes to be our soul, rather than just its window. You can feel the difference between the two states by practising the simply complicated exercise of 'remembering yourself' while placing your awareness in the centre of your being.

Dreamt of a young girl who said, 'You look absolutely lovely.' I knew she meant my whole being rather than my looks.

I dreamt that the mental and emotional characteristics of a person could be understood by looking at their eyes and the surrounding area.

Intellect

Thoughts create a new heaven, a new firmament, a new source of energy, from which new arts flow.

Paracelsus[5]

Neon relates to the brow chakra which governs the intellect.[i] This layer of rationality, numbers, rules and mathematics forms a barrier between us and our higher selves and may prevent us from perceiving the whole truth. Like the iris, the intellect both 'sees' and separates us from reality. Reason is governed by analysis, and therefore division, which both explains and separates us from the all-encompassing oneness of being.

I felt angry and tricked. This all too 'brave new world' was too cheerful and involved deceit.

Mistakes in words. Mistaking 'left' for 'right' and looking at a table and wanting to say 'chair' but saying 'table' instead. The visual stimulus affects my ability to say the right word. Before, the mistakes were closer. Now there is a bigger gap between the word I want and the word I say.

According to a Jewish legend, while we are in the uterus we know all and everything about heaven and earth. The moment we are born, an angel presses his finger to our upper lip, forming the cleft between lip and nose (*the philtral dimple*). At that moment we forget all we that we know. We gain reason and lose knowing. We move from the unified perception of the third eye down to the reason-based mind as seen through our two eyes, from synthesis to analysis. As yet these eyes have not learnt to work in unison. Stereophonic perception appears in Argon and until then the world will remain flat. This flatness may manifest in Neon cases as an overactive intellect or power of reasoning that overrides emotions, for example in cases of Asperger's syndrome, in particular when there is an obsession with numbers.

Skin

References to both physical and metaphoric skin abound in Neon. Along-side the many references to skin and itching we find the following:

---

[i] While the chakras are generally listed from the first chakra in the root to the 7th in the crown, I find that with the noble gases this is reversed, so that the crown chakra is first and relates to Helium, Neon to the brow etc.

This is not really real, It's very much on the surface. It feels skin-deep, on the skin only.

Dreamt I saw the doctor medicate and peel entire skin off the back of the child.

Then I had an image of the inside of a body. I was in the dark but it was bright, like an amazing landscape. . . . 'Epithelium' came to mind.

Skin is surface; epithelial tissue covers the whole surface of the body. It is made up of cells closely packed and arranged in one or more layers. This tissue is specialised to form the covering or lining of all internal and external body surfaces. Epithelial tissue, regardless of its type, is usually separated from the underlying tissue by a thin sheet of connective tissue, basement membrane. Epidermis is a special type of epithelium forming the outer layer of skin. Thus epithelium is an analogue to firmament, the dividing layer which separates our internal and external environments.

Estranged

Finally, the firmament separates us from each other, dividing the oneness of being into in-divi-duals. From:

Overwhelming sensation of being surrounded by love.

The feeling of family went beyond my family to include the entire human race.

To:

I felt alone and as if everyone perceived me as odd. I felt strange, like an outsider and could not connect on any level.

One of our visitors went out to buy a newspaper. When he came back I could not recognise him, although I've known him for 12 years, thinking he was a total stranger.

Living behind our perceived barriers, we become less aware of the big picture and more focused on ourselves.

Somehow I had a very profound realisation that this was my own life time. My usual feelings of guilt shifted and I was able to take responsibility for my own life. During the proving, I wore my glasses more frequently and had dreams of windows. As though there had been a shift of focus to my own needs.

Summary

My prior speculation regarding the relationship between the noble gases and the biblical seven days of creation was confirmed in Helium and again in the proving of Neon. The second day seems to discuss water, but this is not its main subject. God does not create water on the second day, as it already exists on the first day. On the second day the firmament is created, the first barrier. To gain a deeper understanding of Neon, we must study the nature of firmament in all its manifestations (Figure 8.6). In our investigation we have related the firmament to all things that separate: windows, doors, the iris, the skin and the intellect. Neon experiences the expectant desire to penetrate these barriers, to peep through the keyhole to the other side.

Water is the basis of all life and within the watery Neon new life is born. Water creates the homogenous fluidity of existence, as it has no distinguishing features and always looks the same. It lends us the flexibility to mould and adapt to every circumstance by taking the shape of its vessel, and vessels are made of barriers. As newborn babies our identity dissolves and merges with others', but as we grow we form the membranes which envelop

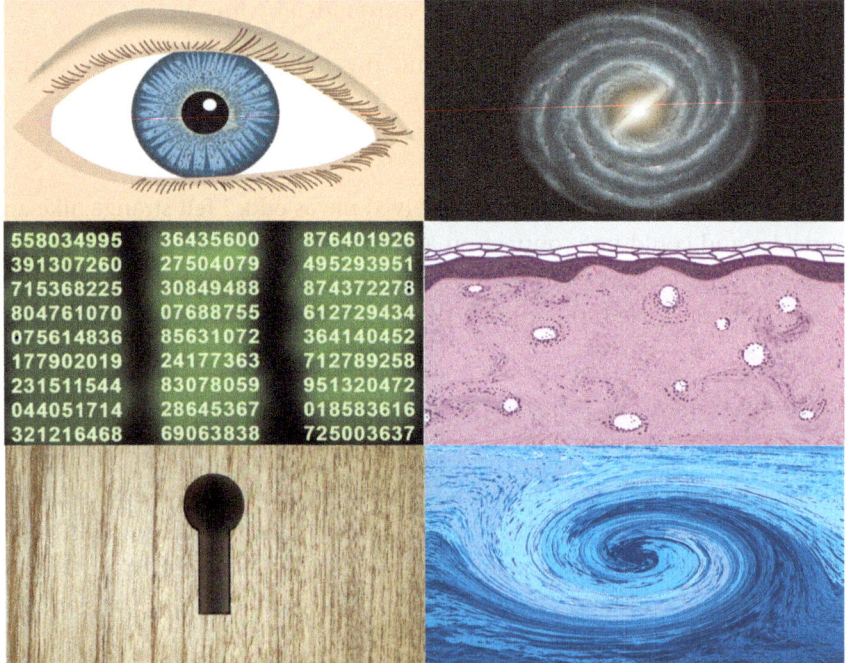

Figure 8.6 *Analogies of the firmament in Neon (clockwise from upper right): galaxy, skin, waters, keyhole, matrix, iris*

and contain our being, giving us our own, separate identity. We may therefore relate the firmament to the high surface tension of water, that which enables water to form individual drops, in other words shapes the sea of souls into soul droplets. This surface tension results in capillary action, representing our ability to rise.

The seeds of our soul originate in the Hydrogen collective soul, which lies beyond the distant stars. But once on earth we must create a distinctive self. The firmament that separates us from our collective roots also divides us from each other and allows us to develop individuality. Each individual is gifted with a magical uniqueness, but this gift comes at a price: potential estrangement, selfishness and desire.

In Chapter 14, I discuss the chemical composition of the firmament.

References

1   Einstein A. Emmy Noether Professor Einstein Writes in Appreciation of a Fellow-Mathematician. *New York Times* May 5, 1935.
2   Bill Murray. Twitter feed. Available online at: https://twitter.com/BilIMurray/status/339759173145350144
3   Tzu L. *Tao Te Ching* (trans Addis S, Lombardo S). Cambridge MA: Hackett Publishing Inc, 1993.
4   Genesis 1:6–8 Bible Gateway. Available online at: https://www.biblegateway.com/passage/?search=Genesis+1:6–8
5   Paracelsus *Quotes*. Available online at: http://historymedren.about.com/od/quotes/a/quote_paracelsu.htm
6   *The Matrix*. Village Roadshow Pictures, 1999.

9

NEON 50M SENSATION, FUNCTION, STRUCTURE

The electric energy which motivates us is not within our bodies at all. It is a part of the universal supply which flows through us from the Universal Source with an intensity set by our desires and our will.

Walter Russell[1]

We now leave the emotional realm and ascend the potencies of perception to the 50M, which relates to the sensations and functions of the remedy. I call this level 'the verb', as it depicts the relative motion of bodies in space and the patterns they create.[i] This level also encompasses the geometrical structure of the remedy. In the following chapter, the proving of Neon will demonstrate how our physical, mental and moral alignment with the universal source directly affects the way we live our life, and conversely, how the various angles which we incline away from it create our pathology.

Window of the sky

It is apparent that while some Neon provers were weak, lethargic, miserable and discontent, others enjoyed clarity, bliss, effortless grace and an endless supply of energy.

Walking was effortless, light and free, I had a sensation of walking uniformly. I feel so different in my body.

Walking up a long gradual incline, I felt I was covering great distances with every stride.

I got busy with building – had masses of energy, felt I could do the impossible.

---

[i] For more information on this method of analysis, see Sherr J. *Dynamic Materia Medica – Syphilis* (2nd edn). Glasgow: Saltire Books, 2014.

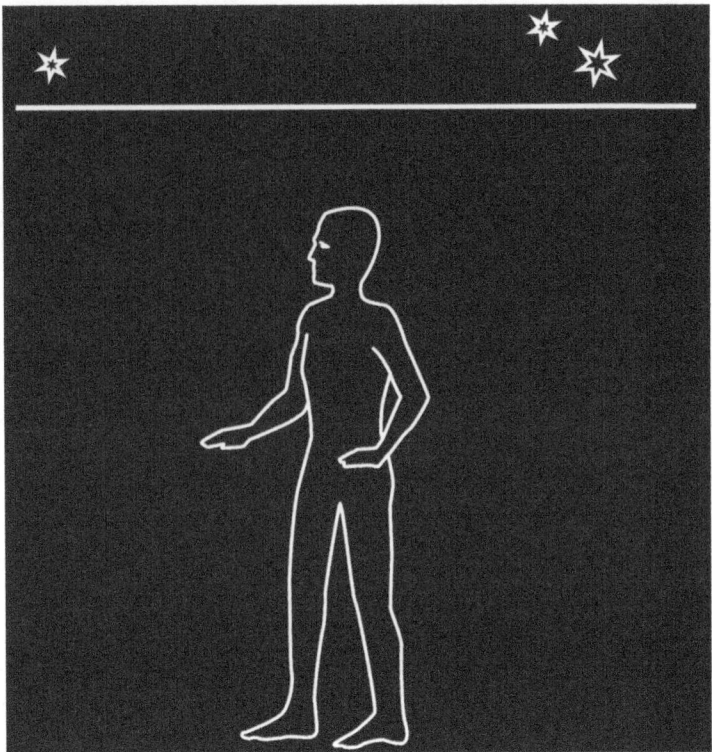

Figure 9.1 Separated from heaven by the firmament

Under what conditions can Neon experience this incredible power? Usually the firmament prevents us from receiving limitless universal energy. Like a membrane covering our being, the firmament stops us from reconnecting to the source. Anything that prevents the Force from flowing may be considered a firmament; barriers such as the sky, clouds, the skull, the iris and most especially human logic obstruct the free flow of heavenly energy. Like Bob Dylan's song, *Knockin' on Heaven's Door,* written for the soundtrack of the film *Pat Garrett and Billy the Kid* (MGM 1973), we long for a crack in the firmament, a gap through which we can reconnect and receive heavenly energy (Figure 9.1). Neon, newly born into the 'real' world and acutely aware of this firmament, longs to penetrate the barriers that separate us from the heavens and somehow reconnect to universal energy.

I just long for some clear nights so I can see my stars. If I could reconnect, then everything would be all right.

I had intense pleasure at hearing the wind and I thought, 'It will clear the skies.'

If this firmament could be penetrated, if we could only find an opening, all heaven would break loose. And somehow, at some point, Neon breaks through.

Felt wonderful. At last the sky was clear, moon brilliant, stars familiar, air cold. I felt so much a part of everything again.

Looking out of the window at the night sky, it suddenly cracked open and a great darkness revealed itself.

Image of being inside my iris and I was looking through it. From the centre of it light was radiating out.

While looking at a star map it looked unfamiliar, as if I had always been seeing the stars from the other side.

Once the barrier is penetrated, we can enjoy unbounded universal energy rather than being dependent on our own pathetic and limited supply. Like a Jedi tuning into 'the Force', we align ourselves with the gap in the firmament so that pure power can permeate our being and ignite our light sabres.

I have superbly fluid and graceful motions, as if I were moving in water instead of air.

On walking in the fresh air, I suddenly felt as if I was cruising along on an energy which was not of my own muscular power. It seemed as if it was

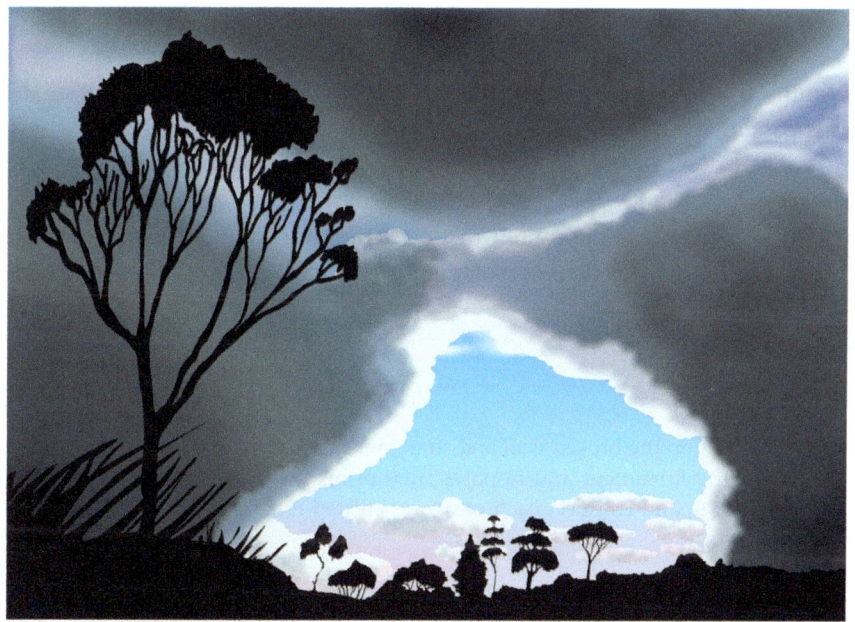

Figure 9.2 Window of the sky

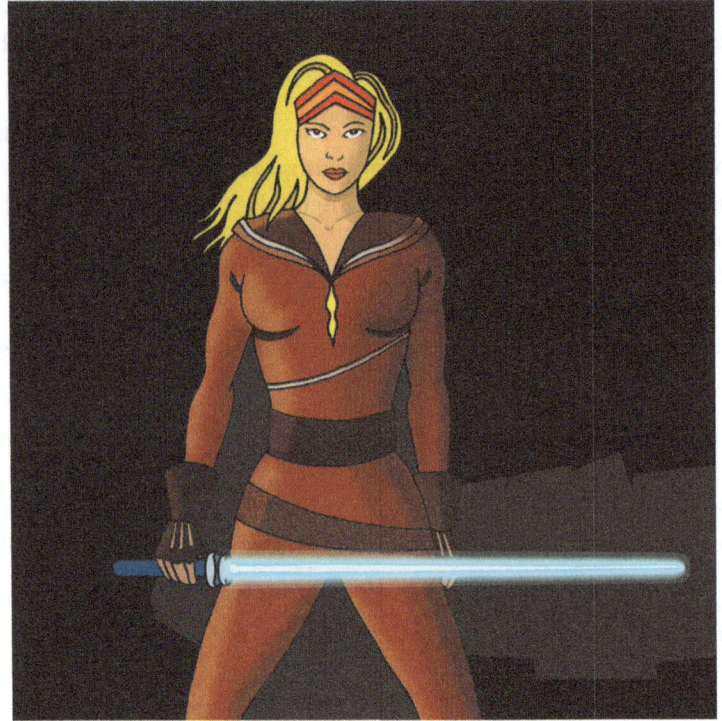

Figure 9.3 Jedi with light sabre

coming from somewhere else. It seemed effortless and unreal. I felt as if I was passing everyone else.

Looked down at my feet and thought they looked really healthy and glowing.

Lay in bed and my body felt insubstantial, starting with my hands and forearms – as if I was dematerialising, 'beaming down.'

Upright

> Love builds up the broken wall and straightens the crooked path. Love keeps the stars in the firmament and imposes rhythm on the ocean tides. Each of us is created of it, and I suspect each of us was created for it.
>
> Maya Angelou[2]

How does Neon achieve this amazing state of grace, in which it receives energy directly from above? The answer must be that there is a 'window in the sky', a gap in the barrier through which universal energy 'The Force'

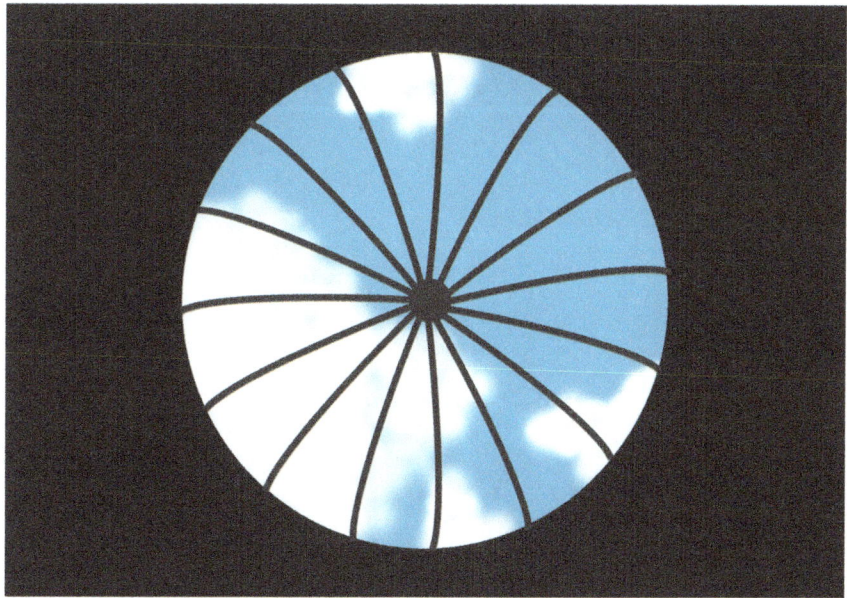

Figure 9.4 *Window to the sky*

can freely flow (Figure 9.4). But where is this window and how can we access it? I will demonstrate that this window is located directly above us, a vertical vortex to our vertex. Notice the location of the window in the following symptom.

My head above my eyes cleared. It felt like a very **wide opening from the top of my head outwards**. I felt a total synchronicity. I didn't have to get to a thought, bring it up, act. I was observing the mechanics of thoughts instead of needing them. It was effortless. While I felt I wasn't having thoughts, I was still doing everything that I usually do. Everything was more beautiful. There was total order in space, more stability.

The window is always there, directly above us. To receive universal energy we must align ourselves with it, make a small adjustment in our physical and spiritual posture. In other words, we need to be upright! (Figure 9.5)

I feel invincible when upright. No wavering – like a laser.

I now feel very upright in space and am aware that before, I was at a slight tilt – both physically and morally. The whole proving can be described as a rectification.

A weight has been lifted, the bowed feeling has been replaced by upright-ness.

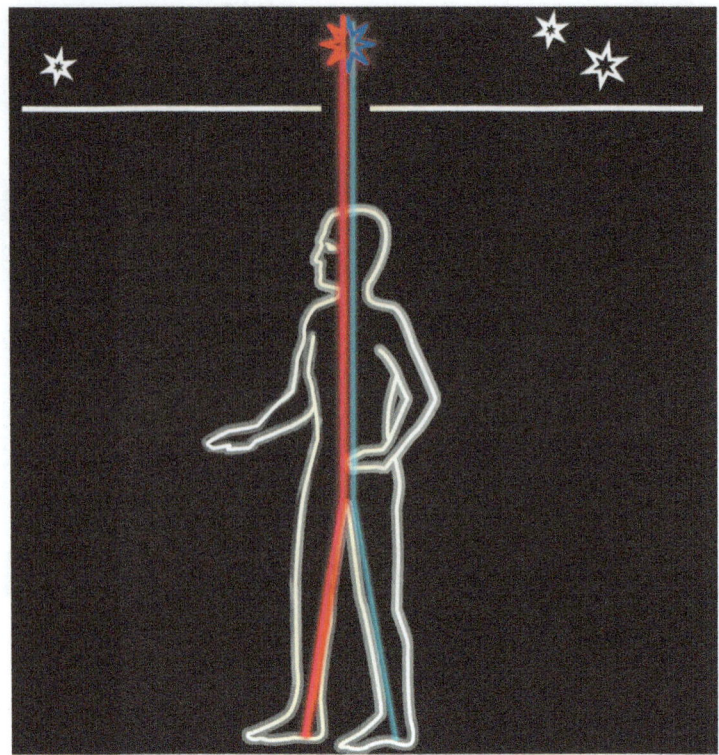

Figure 9.5 When we line up with the sky window we are blessed with heavenly energy

Once we are aligned, there is no stopping the energy, spiritual power or bliss of heaven.

I feel more stable now that my feet touch the earth while my head still touches the heavens.

Feel like I have been kissed by heaven.

Now I feel no resistance, a harmony between heaven and earth.

It was all there in front of me but I felt too unsure to truly see it before. As if a veil had gone.

My head feels so good – supremely coherent.

The upright direction is best depicted by the following symptom:

I kept seeing the image of a circle with an arrow going straight up from the top of it. I was aware of the circle but I could not see the centre of it. My awareness remained focused on the arrow. (Figure 9.6)

If we lean forwards into the future, backwards into the past, or sideways into desire, selfishness or logic, we lose the connection and tilt into the

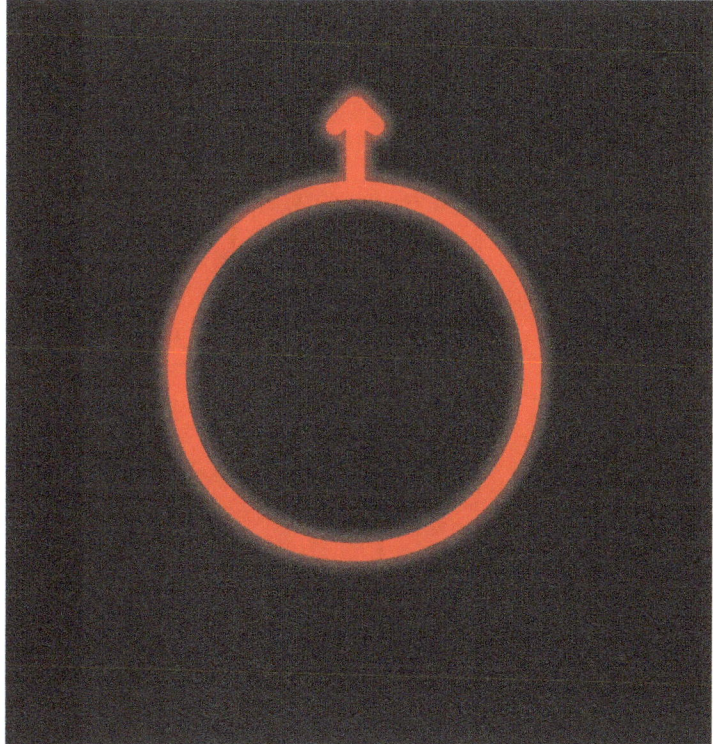

Figure 9.6 Vertical connection

muck and mire of earthly dependence (Figure 9.7). It is only by the rectification of our being that we can align with the universal force.

Slight light-headedness when reading with my head leaning forward, better when I lift my head so that my spine is straight, better when I fix my eyes in the distance.

My spirit feels light without being weightless. Prior to taking the remedy, I felt too far in the future, without realising it. I feel as if I have taken a step back and am in the here and now.

Doing research on Uranus, I found that the planet has a tilt. For 42 years one side is in the dark and then it comes into the light for 42 years.

When we are upright, the membranes which occlude our being are penetrated and the waters of life can truly flow, cerebral spinal fluid traversing our brain (Figure 9.8).

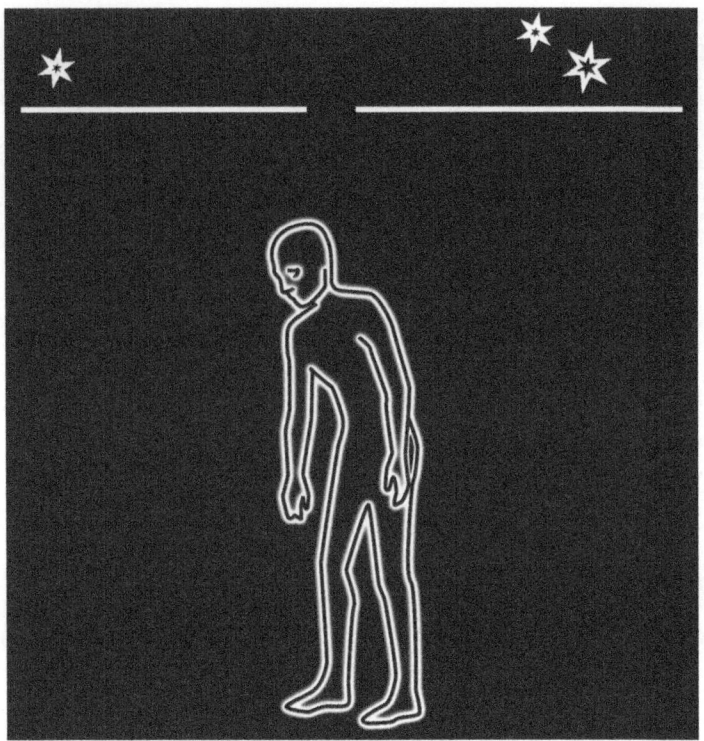

Figure 9.7 *When we are not upright we no longer align with the Source*

The following was quoted on page 37 in another context.

A phrase from a Lewis Carroll poem[3] repeated itself over and over in my mind:

> I saw an aged, aged man,
> A-sitting on a gate.
> "Who are you, aged man?" I said,
> "And how is it you live?"
> And his answer trickled through my head,
> Like water through a sieve.

I felt this was about dissolving, which related to my feeling during the proving.

'And how is it you live?' The upright position pertains to our whole being, physically, mentally and morally. As long as we lean into a divided life we remain dependent upon our own fuel and on terrestrial resources, depleting ourselves and our planet. Everything becomes an effort. Our internal firmament divides our existence and leaves in its wake the barriers of time, the number Two, desires and logic, all of which obscure our true potential.

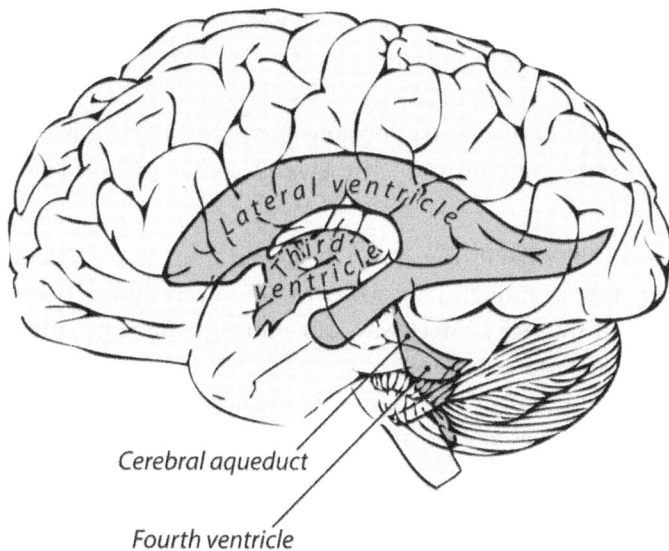

Cerebral aqueduct

Fourth ventricle

Figure 9.8 *The brain*

To reconnect with unlimited universal resources, we must align with the window in the sky and receive energy directly from heaven. This alignment depends on reuniting the two sides of our being and eliminating the constraints of desire. In the upright state, in the here and now, Neon rests in the bliss of the eternal moment, floating effortlessly on the rivers of time. When the window on top of our heads is directly aligned with the window in the sky, we are open to the heavenly lakes of wisdom, the waters of the sky.

This is the secret of the noble Neon.

Walking was effortless, light and free, with a sensation of walking uniformly. I feel so different in my body. I am all in the now, especially in my lower legs and feet. At last, I touch the earth. I now feel forgiven for the ultimate sin. I feel unbounded love for myself but I wonder, 'Is there a "me" anymore?' No more separations!

Angles of the periodic table

Materia Medica never inspires perception. The physician must have the love of its use, and he becomes wise in proportion as he loves his use, and in proportion as he lives uprightly with his patients; that is, desires to heal them; beautify their souls. Can the physician, who does not love his neighbor as himself, get into this position?

> The upright man, whose desires are good, wants the truth. His perceptions are intensified.
>
> JT Kent[4]

The theme of uprightness versus leaning also occurs in Helium. The following Helium symptoms relate to the idea of seeing oneself from directly above.

> Feels as if I see myself from the outside and from above. (Helium)
>
> Feel very tall, as though I am towering over everything. (Helium)
>
> I see myself in a very direct way, as if from the outside, with no holds barred. I feel superior. (Helium)
>
> Sense that all limbs are foreshortened, my head and eyes feel huge, I feel as though I have eyes all over my head, that I am all-seeing. (Helium)

The theme of being both large and small is repeated in Neon.

> After a shower, I felt enormous, massive, yet in proportion. I was amazed at how huge I was.
>
> I felt as if I had shrunk, particularly my legs. My legs felt shorter.

This sensation, of being tall with short limbs, is shared by the first two noble gas remedies. Only by viewing from above along a vertical line running through the body can one gain such a perspective. Helium views the body directly from overhead so that they feel tall while the body appears foreshortened. The Helium dilemma is whether to remain in the pristine world of souls above or whether to lean forward and make the leap into the terrestrial world below. Only once they lean will they develop a shadow side, the duality of life. Neon is positioned lower down along this line so that the emphasis is on shorter legs. When Neon is aligned in its central position there is no division of time or space. Neon's dilemma is whether to remain central and upright or whether to tilt forwards or backwards and be ruled by time and its consequent desires.

The concept of being upright and aligned is a 'family trait' of the noble gases, repeating in several of the group VIII remedies. In contrast, the 'ordinary' elements lean at various angles to the vertical axis of existence (Figure 9.9). They seek to rectify themselves to the perpendicular but can only do so by means of chemical interactions, in which they share electrons to mimic the noble uprightness.

By studying the meaning of each noble gas's rectification, as achieved through vertical alignment, we can perceive its true nature and understand what the preceding period yearns for. Hydrogen, in the first period, lies in a horizontal line. Spread across the universe and with no focus, it has lost its connection with the collective soul; therefore, it yearns to regain

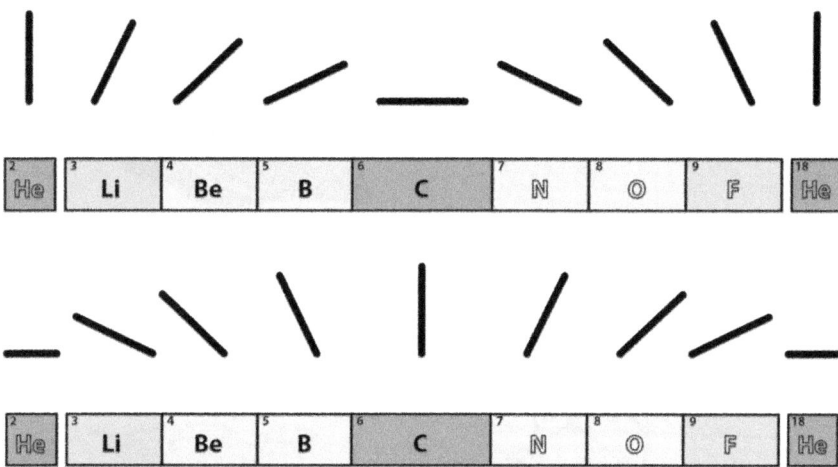

Figure 9.9 Angles of the periodic table. The top diagram shows upright nobles while the bottom has them in an inert state

purpose through aligning itself with the individual, upright mission of Helium. Helium, however, is stuck in this vertical prison, unable to lean forward into life.

Each element or remedy holds within it the opposite and perpendicular state.

Dream we went into an auditorium to see some kind of lecture or theatre, and sat in the front row, but the chairs were at a 90 degree angle to the stage.

The bottom diagram in Figure 9.9 shows the opposite, perpendicular state inherent in each remedy. At their worst the noble gases become inert and prostrate, lying horizontally and thus cut off from universal energy and the purpose of life. Here, Helium and Neon are shown in their flat state, as opposed to the aligned and electrified position in the top diagram.

Carbon, the middle element of the series, is shown as inert and flat in the top diagram (Graphites), but is in an upright noble state in the bottom diagram (Adamas). The periodic wave has reversed polarity.

Graphite and diamond are both allotropes of carbon. As a result of their distinct crystal structures they have different properties (Figure 9.10). Graphite has a **two-dimensional** lattice structure of horizontal layers of carbon atoms.[5] Whilst the atoms in each layer are held together by strong covalent bonds, the bonds between each layer, which are stacked on top of each other, are relatively weak. Hence, graphite is soft, slippery and black; its hardness is less than one on the Mohs scale. Graphite can be used as a

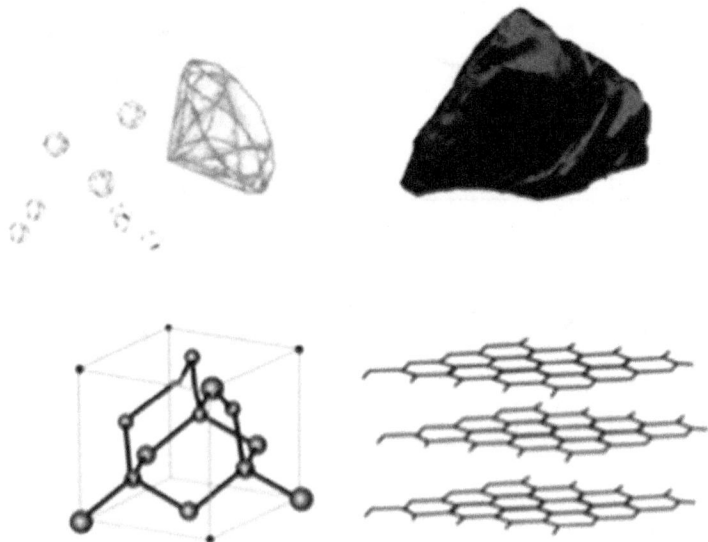

Figure 9.10 The structures of diamond and graphite

lubricant or in pencils because the layers slide easily. In contrast, diamond has a strong, rigid **three-dimensional** tetrahedral structure. Hence it is the hardest material known – 10 on the Mohs scale. The brilliant diamond shines by refracting and dispersing light, and is a powerful conductor of heat.

The difference between the phlegmatic, soft and lazy Graphites and the brilliant, noble Adamas is a result of their respective two or three dimensional arrangement. These three spatial dimensions, line, surface and volume, unfold in the first three periods, as we transition from Helium to Neon and beyond. This dimensional relationship to the periodic table is examined in Chapter 10, 'New Dimensions'.

Meditation provings on remedies of the second period

The angular attitudes of the elements as illustrated in Figure 9.9 are apparent in their full proving pictures as well as in several single-blind mini-meditation provings from my wife Camilla (*in italics*).[i]

As can be seen in Figure 9.9, the elemental remedies of the second period, Lithium to Fluoride, lean into various angles from the vertical, and are inclined at 22.5° (180° divided by 8) off each other: 90°, 77.5°, 55°, 22.5°

---

[i] The full transcripts of Camilla's provings will be published in the future.

and 0°. These angles signify aspects of space, time, desire and rationality; the elements' susceptibility to the slanted world of reality. They strive to emulate the best of Helium or Neon by re-aligning vertically, but they can only become upright by combining with other elements. We therefore study each of these elements in this context.

The top diagram shows the almost vertical slant of Lithium and Fluoride. These 'almost there' angles lend great reactivity to both these elements. In contrast, Beryllium, and especially Boron, are on their way down (*fear of downward motion*), while Nitrogen and Oxygen are gaseous and hence have an upward motion.

In the bottom diagram, which is perpendicular to the top diagram, we see Lithium in an almost horizontal angle (*My lower lip wants to turn inside out. It feels all floppy and wants to curl outwards and down*).

Beryllium

We find baby Beryllium lifting his head for the first time and taking an insecure peek at a bewildering new world, one that is not entirely real and is prone to collapse at any time.

This is like a Hollywood Halloween, not the real thing, like a joke, like a cartoon but different. Like a facade, Disney world, you make it scary but it is not really. Like it's empty behind. Like Orlando – facade with no substance, just an act, make believe. This feels not one ounce real. A gust of wind, a creaky gate, empty clichés that should evoke something in you.

Like a 4 or 5 year old. Someone who plays 'home' with a make-believe cookery set. The stage where you are scared of vampires, you don't know what is real and not. Playing pretend play: Let's pretend this is a saloon, that this is a cooker, that I'm cooking food for you now. Let's pretend you are in little house in the prairie. Don't know what is real and what is not. Are monsters real, is Halloween real? Before the comprehending stage. Like being scared of clowns because you don't know what is behind it, a mask. A bit eerie. You haven't quite made sense of the world yet. You are a kid. The age where you're trying to make sense of the world. Or not even trying yet. It's just copying. I see my mum cooking so now I'm cooking like that. Not asking why. It is the copying stage, mimicking. Not creating. Mimic copy. Like reflex stage, like learning to play tennis, copy at the beginning.

Boron

Another example of the contrast between these two perpendicular angles can be seen in the following mini-meditation proving of Boron from Camilla. Boron, which was nearly falling in the top diagram, is now rising to almost vertical, like a toddler transforming from crawling to walking, struggling to grow a physical and mental 'spine' and stand upright.

This remedy is emotional. A heaviness is descending on me. Heavy feeling – (Observation – she is making a downward motion over head till shoulders. Corners of mouth going down in a frown. Pulling them down with hand.) I feel really, really fat. I am a fat, heavy, pathetic disgusting being. Yuck. Self hatred and self loathing, I'm gross. Like I'm really fat, huge fat body, gross, stomach huge, gross and ugly. Going horizontal like fat goo. Face growing sideways. Image from a movie: Like Meryl Streep movie (devil something) where they turn their heads around. Like rubber. Feel gross, like a toad. Face pulled out sideways. Want to remold face.

Now that's finished! Now I'm the opposite, all thin, puckering lips in. Now all thin and body sucked in, together, tight, firm and thin and upright. And with muscle tone. I feel my cheeks being pulled in. Before I was all splat horizontal outwards, like someone splat me, now opposite being sucked in. The answer is to be upright so that you can't be flattened. I feel I could dislocate my vertebra and own neck. Weird body sensation. I felt elongating and changing shape. Like a funny mirror, like Alice in Wonderland. As if I am made from rubber. When you are thin you are in control. All tight and in control, as opposed to fat and all over the place and self loathing fat blubber rolling all over you. I can really feel my spine. I can feel my spine all the way down. I am sharp and focused and together and tight and controlled. Like being horizontal vs. being vertical. Must control the rubbery body. When I'm upright I feel my spine, I have got one. But when the opposite, no spine, you just expand horizontally. Fear of being the blubbery, fat piece of lard. This would be perfect for obsessive compulsives, control freaks, eating disorders. Rubber face, like Jim Carrey.

Having a spine or no spine: spineless describes the fat disgusting thing lying on the sofa with no will power and self loathing. A bit bi-polar on both sides. Eating disorders, go from one to the other. Like an actor getting no parts and feeling a failure. Literally can't pull yourself together. Then you get a part and you pull yourself together, now you have it, in control.

Could be the stage you get your spine as a foetus, but the rest like an immature person, doesn't know who you are yet, trying to make sense of it, being pulled in two directions, fighting between two polarities. Or if someone squashes you and you develop lack of confidence, maybe if you are told that you are no good. Self-confidence squashed, and then you try to pull yourself together to say, ok I'm good. But in this you need help from outside. This remedy is influenced from outside events and people, no spine. Either others approve of you or don't. Like the heaviness that descended on me came from the outside. Or getting a part in the movie depends on the outside. This remedy thrives on outside influence, other people's approval. You are not really your own master. Someone tells you that you are crap or good, that you got the movie part or not, peer pressure. To get out must amalgamate the two together and grow your own spine.

Note: No wonder Boron has a fear of falling (Borax). When it is nearly upright it gains strength and confidence, but when it falls into a spineless state it becomes a helpless toddler who cannot stand on his own feet. While this proving contrasts a vertical and horizontal state, it is also apparent that these two states are not precisely vertical or horizontal, 180° or 90°. Both Boron states are not independent of external influence, as in the noble gases, but rather dependant on others' opinions and support. The slight tilt provides a susceptibility.

Carbon

Carbon sits safely at the cross roads of the centre of the second period. In the top diagram (Figure 9.9) it lies prostrate, in a lethargic horizontal line, while in the bottom diagram it is vertical and noble. From this middle position, and with the help of its four arms it can turn left or right, up or down, to grasp hydrogen, oxygen, nitrogen, sulphur and many other atoms.[3] Hence, carbon provides the structure for the whole organic world. This multidirectional and multifaceted ability also provides its neutrality, making Carbon the 'invisible remedy of the materia medica.' In a proving of pure Carbon by Jurgen Becker, one prover dreamt of a father beating his child through an invisible mother who stood between them. Carbon is the unseen mother, the no-name Mrs. or Dr. John Smith of our materia medica. She has four arms, being the mother, cook, accountant, cleaning lady, lover and taxi driver. She does everything but is never recognised for her efforts, holding the family together and making the world go round. She lives off the opinion of others and is seen only as an extension of her partner. This woman will state her profession as 'Nothing really, I am only a housewife'. These Carbon issues are clearly seen in the proving of Adamas.[6]

Likewise, homoeopaths often make the mistake of ignoring the essential Carbon ion in a remedy, claiming they have given 'Baryta', 'Magnesium' or 'Calcarea', and extrapolating remedy pictures based on these ion bachelors while ignoring the mother. Others claim she is the father, oblivious of the invisible mother behind the man.

In Camilla's remarkable meditation proving of Carbon (once again single blind) the four directional carbon cross can be seen clearly. Here the vertical noble strength opposes the horizontal weakness, all 90° angles. The cross intersects at the neck.

As I have explained in 'The Introduction to the Noble Gases', in *Helium* there is a direct relationship between the central column of the periodic table and the noble gases.[7] The relationship is confirmed and emphasised by this proving, with Carbon showing many similarities to its opposite element Neon. When upright, a huge amount of universal energy comes in through the vertex. When curved the energy is blocked. This is the great secret.

Head lifting up, like beaming upwards. I feel I am being elongated and pulled upwards, as if my head is elongating, up, up, up. Head becoming really long, like a cone. I am being pulled upwards from my head.

I feel strange, like my whole awareness is at the top. I just keep going up, I don't know if it will ever stop.

(Observation: Eyeballs rolling backwards.)

Tingling around crown.

I feel I should be sitting upwards but I can't be bothered. It doesn't matter, still beaming up, a powerful sensation.

I feel out of it, almost drugged, strange sensation.

As if my body is insignificant. Only the head is important, especial top of head.

It's not a cone, more like a funnel, my whole head is opening up.

It's best not to be upright or it will surge though the body. Best to be curved.

The neck is a very fragile point in the body. You have to be very careful with neck, it can break so easily. Make sure the kids always wear belts in the car.

(Observation: Twisting neck around.)

Like my face and jaw are changing. Something coming in and changing the shape of my head and jaw.

(Observation: Sitting very upright, twisting jaw around.)

I feel like I need to turn my head to feel where it is, to do circles with my head so I can feel where its edges are, where the periphery is, how big is it.

(Observation: Turning head and neck in circles.)

Neck feels very stiff.

Feels like a big funnel coming out of my head, when I move my head a whole massive funnel is moving with it. When I bend my head down the funnel moves with it, like I could draw or paint with it.

I get the image of the Pharaoh with his upside down cone-shaped crown.

It is a hat, like a funnel, open at the top.

(Observation: Still turning head up, down, right, left.)

The easiest way to kill someone is to kill their neck. Very fragile, the neck.

I get the sensation you either have to face completely straight forward, or with head totally bent to the side. You can't do angles or degrees, not comfortable. Either full front face, or neck turned 90 degrees.

I feel like a sphinx.

(**Observation:** *Turning head full left, then full right.*)

The funnel is so heavy, it is not good to bend head down, you could topple over. You have to be straight.

I can hear my neck scrunching. The neck feels very thin and delicate.

The funnel is for energy and power and the connection upwards. It forces you to be upright, like I didn't want to be upright but I had to.

Don't want to pull this energy into my body, just shut it in the head.

I don't know what to do with all this energy. I don't know if to let it in through the neck. What if it doesn't get out. What if the funnel closes and it gets trapped inside me.

I feel if I could stand up and I could do anything.

I could do sorcery, very powerful energy.

(**Observation:** *She stands up.*)

I could just go Poccchhhh (stamping foot). I now feel this energy going right through my body. (Observation: Stamping hard.)

I could set things on fire with my hands. Energy surging though my arms.

(**Observation:** *Walking very upright with head straight. Puffing out forcefully while stamping foot and jerking hands downwards.*)

Pooofff! Very strong energy through body. This is really powerful!!

A huge surge of energy, tingling all though my body, electricity. Emitting a huge amount of power. Like one of the heroes in the TV series' Hero' or an 'X man', I just wave my hand and fire or sparks come out, electricity. My hands are completely warm – very unusual, they were freezing before.

Tingling all over my body, all over my legs.

Again the elongation and opening in head.

I feel like the letter C, bent over. I need to be straight.

I feel quite indifferent, detached.

I feel very powerful, like a ruler, a king. A magician or a king, very high up.

Like huge power and you just do 'Phoo' and it will happen.

You can make the cone bigger and smaller with the rotation of your head, little or big circles. Control the amount of energy coming in.

Turning neck 90 degrees left and right. Now I can turn it without any problems.

Before elbow hurt, now right knee hurting a bit.

I never experienced anything like this in my life.

(**Observation:** *Standing straight, hands spread and fingers spread down, and beginning to cry and sigh deeply. Crying and sighing.*

Stomping the ground. Deep sighs.)

Wow!! Thank you!

I feel so huge, like a massive amount of energy surging through my body and cleaning it out, a huge release, I don't know of what. Every muscle in my body was tensing and now releasing through. I feel like crying but I don't know why.

Wow. It would take 50 years of yoga and meditation to get what I just got. I'll never be the same again.

All energy going through me, I am so connected my feet are completely on the ground. My toes and fingers spread out. Eternal life, if you let it flow and don't block it. We are just all the time blocking it, all the time, resisting it. It's just there for everybody.

We are not aware and no one ever taught us how to do that.

Open it up and leave it open and let it all in. It's really important. We must not limit ourselves, we put limitations, but there are no limitations at all, they don't exist. Limitations come from blocking the energy and not letting it pass through.

My neck is completely free.

All the suppression, everything is gone. Everything stored in my body and muscles is released. I released so much, every emotion that was stored in my muscles and physical body, all are washed out and released. That is why I was crying. I could feel every muscle, muscles I did not know existed, all released. I feel lifetimes of baggage all out. Now it's going into the ground.

Wow! What a present, Oh my God. Thank you.

I feel so humbled and unworthy of this! I feel like God went through my body.

Crying. I feel unworthy of this present, it's too big. But I am not going to block it. Just say thank you to God.

Sighing deeply.

A feeling of freedom, No limitations, so much abundance. You don't need to struggle for money, just open up and it will rain on you. (Observation: Laughing.) Anything is possible. I realise that I was just creating limitation for myself. Limiting myself. I can do anything.

Just release the energy, let go the struggle, the hardship, limitations, problems, all preconceived ideas. Just think of the dream and focus and what you want. Just a matter of wanting it and it will come, you create it. See your dream, not the difficulties, let it go into the ground, power your body and think of what you want and it cannot not come.

I feel my face has relaxed for the first time ever.

I feel i gained a million years of wisdom. Connecting. Seeing connections, like little lights going on everywhere, all my thoughts connecting. I can create! I can make, I can do, it will happen.

I think when you die you have it like that. Your soul soars and you are free completely.

It's a Tikun (Cabbalistic rectification)

A massive ripple effect all over. I feel like the whole planet is correcting itself, the people connected to me.

Like the grand cross in the sky right now.

And down the line

Following on from Carbon we find Nitrogen veering off centre (*very aware of the curve of my body slouching, not straight, I should be sitting up*). Oxygen, lying midway between vertical and horizontal at 45°, is prone to alternating up and down moods. Similarly Ozone dreams of descending up and down a mountain. Fluoride is almost prostrate with weakness.

Further discussions on Fluorine, Oxygen and Ozone can be found in Chapter 14.

References

1   Russell W. *Inspirational Quotes.* https://www.entheos.com/quotes/by_teacher/walter+russell

2   Angelou M. Available online at: http://www.spiritual-blog.com/tag/quotes-on-love/

3   A poem by Lewis Carroll from *Through the Looking-Glass*. It is sung by The White Knight in Chapter eight to a tune that he claims as his own invention, but which Alice recognises as "I give thee all, I can no more". Available online at: http://www.poemhunter.com/poem/the-aged-aged-man/comments/

4   Kent JT. The trend of thought necessary for the comprehension and retention of the application of the homoeopathic materia medica in New Remedies, Clinical Cases, *Lesser Writings, Aphorisms and Precepts*. New Delhi, India: B. Jain Publishers Pvt. Ltd, 1998, p. 647, 656.

5   *Why is Graphite soft and Diamond hard if both are pure carbon?* The Interactive Library. Available online at: http://www.edinformatics.com/interactive molecules/graphite.htm

6   Sherr J. *Dynamis Provings Volume I.* Malvern: Dynamis Books, 1997.

7   Sherr J. *Dynamic Materia Medica: Helium.* Glasgow: Saltire Books, 2013.

10

NEON CM COLLECTIVE SPIRITUALITY

New dimensions

> Our soul is cast into a body, where it finds number, time, dimension. Thereupon it reasons, and calls this nature necessity, and can believe nothing else.
>
> Blaise Pascal[1]

In my exploration of the noble gases I have found that each of the periods creates a new dimension in the space-time continuum. This evolution begins with the singularity of the pre-hydrogen state in which all dimensions are compressed into one. Helium unfolds the first dimension, a line (Figure 10.1). A line has only one dimension because only one coordinate is needed to specify the location of a point on the line (for example, the point with coordinate 5 on a numbered line). As mentioned in the first book of this series, we can assume that the Helium line is oriented vertically because of the many references to feeling tall, to ascending and descending, to high places, to mountains and to viewing the world from above. The direction of the first line is subject to different points of view, as we will later see, but for now we will remain with the vertical Helium.

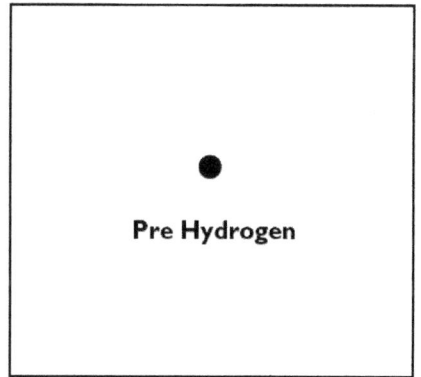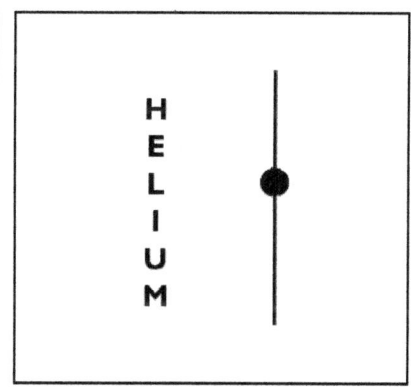

Figure 10.1 Pre-hydrogen singularity unfolding into the first dimension of Helium line

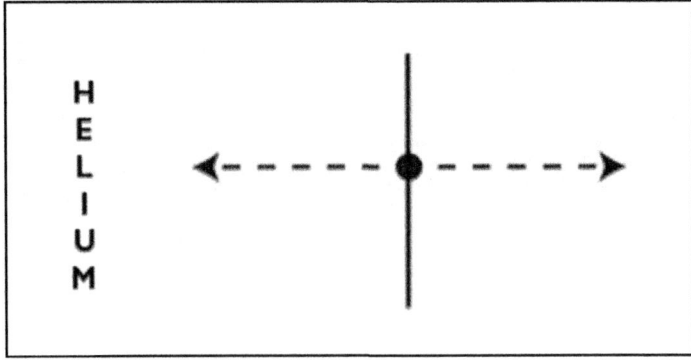

Figure 10.2 Helium's vertical direction creates susceptibility to width

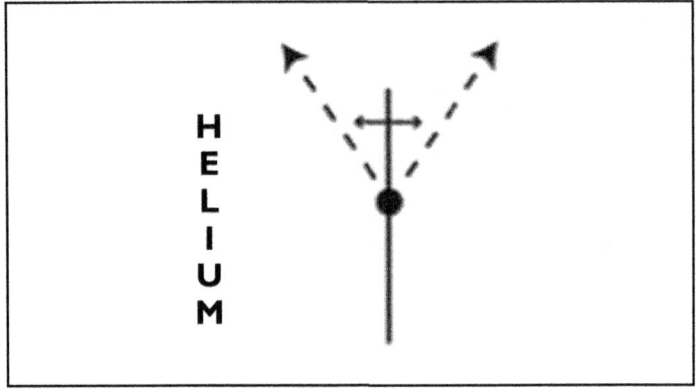

Figure 10.3 Line splitting into two. New direction begins to manifest

By manifesting height, Helium's vertical line creates the possibility of a left-right division (Figure 10.2). This presents a susceptibility to the second period, which will stretch into a new direction – width.

To manifest into this new direction, Helium must split out of its line-prison by dividing into two and tilting.[i] (Figure 10.3). This unfolds within the second period.

As this spilt continues to expand and widen, it becomes perpendicular to the vertical, creating width. This division is completed in Neon; the new line lies horizontally, separating above from below, a firmament (Figure 10.4).

---

[i] For an illustration of this concept please see Case 8.2 'Starry Night'. In: Sherr J. *Dynamic Materia Medica: Helium.* Glasgow: Saltire Books, 2013. p. 90.

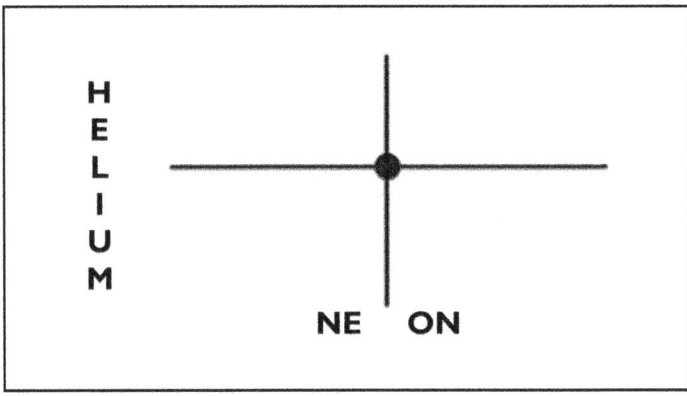

Figure 10.4 *Width unfolds*

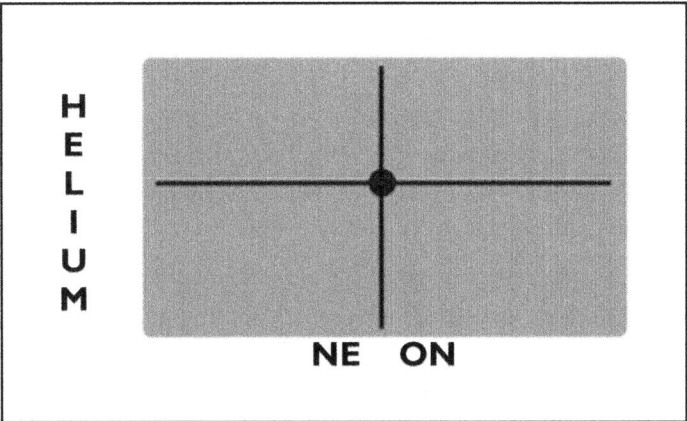

Figure 10.5 *The perpendicular lines of Helium and Neon create surface*

Previously, I described Neon's relationship to the number two as a division. Now this number takes on a new significance, this time as a multiplier, the creator of a new dimension.

Occasional thoughts about numbers: I had always felt comfortable with odd numbers. Now, being both gave a **whole other dimension.**

By manifesting a new line at 90° to Helium, the second period, culminating in Neon, creates a new direction that results in a new dimension – line squared, line^2 or surface (Figure 10.5).

A surface has two dimensions because two coordinates are needed to specify points in its plane (longitude and latitude). Thus, Neon deals with planes, such as firmaments, water surfaces, doors, windows, the skin and the iris. In this shallow world it can play with the geometry of shape, forming angles. It can align with Helium's vertical axis, lean into the future or the past, desires or aversions. It can peek through keyholes. Neon lives on a surface and is a prisoner of its two-dimensional world. It is interesting to read the following from a case of a boy with Attention Deficit Disorder.[ii]

The boy's muscular system was generally highly hypotonic. His mouth was always slightly open and his coordination defective. He often stumbled; he had to touch everything, and was unable to carry out any cross-coordination. Furthermore, he had problems conceiving positions and measurements in three-dimensional space. This was, for example, displayed by the fact that he couldn't crawl underneath tables or chairs without getting stuck because he would perceive a supposed obstacle due to his false bodily conception.

Understanding the development of dimensions in the context of the periodic table has given me a new tool for analyzing cases. If I can perceive the dimension in which a patient is trapped, I may gain insight into a case and remedies needed.

It is interesting to note that other elements in the second period also display two-dimensional issues (see Chapter 9 Angles of the Periodic Table). One example would be the graphites two-dimensional structure versus the diamond three-dimensional structure. Another example is from my proving of Ozone.

I was standing beside this woman who's holding her baby. We're talking and it's friendly. We're looking, facing a mountain in front of us, but it's like a drawing. It's not real looking. There was a bit of 2D quality to it. (Ozone, JS)

The two-dimensional nature of Neon's personality manifests as emotional immaturity. Like a baby, Neon may vacillate between simple emotions of bliss and wretchedness, content and discontent, tranquillity and anxiety, selfishness and gratitude.

As the periods and dimensions unfold we gain some degrees of freedom and lose others. On one hand, Helium is a soul free from physical constraints, while Neon is confined to the prison of life in a body. On the other hand, Neon has more freedom than the one-dimensional Helium, who is confined to a narrow line of existence that is defined in simple binary terms as incarnate or remain in the world of souls, light or darkness, yes or no, clean or dirty. Neon can thus navigate the surface of a two-dimensional world that Helium cannot yet imagine.

[ii] See Chapter 12, Case 12.11: Attention deficit (hyperactivity) disorder.

Neon craves the next, third, dimension of volume or space, and seeks to evolve into it by waiting for a knock on the door or a window to open. Spying through the keyhole of its captive surface, Neon waits for the shell to crack, for relationships to gel, for sperm to penetrate ova. However, unfolding into the third dimension is beyond its reach and Neon remains trapped in its child-like world. It seeks depth but cannot perceive or understand it. The evolution into the complex emotional world of a teenager will not happen until the next period, Sodium to Argon.

Felt like a child – enjoying.

I notice a foolish and irresistible desire to spy on my partner through the keyhole of the door to his study. I am finding it ridiculous, laughing to myself. I feel like a **mischievous child doing something he shouldn't do**, giggling away to myself. It makes me feel **excited in a childish sense**.

The book *Flatland*[3] offers an excellent exploration of the concept of dimensions. A summary is presented in Chapter 14 'Analogy, cosmology, biology'.

The Periodic slide – Dimensions unfolding

No-thing was every-where. No-thing was every-time.
No-thing was bored.
No-thing decided to pack up its no-things
And go no-where else
But it left some-thing:
A dot.

.

Dot was every-thing
Every-thing was dot.
Dot looked around.
There was no-thing to be seen.

Dot tried to move up.
Dot tried to move sideways.
Dot tried to move forward.
It could not. It was dot.

Man, this was frustrating.
Dot could not take it much longer.
Dot got all en-tangled with itself
The pressure was building fast

Dot was getting mad, real mad
Dot was about to expl-!
Bang.
Dot was free!

It was heaven, it was bliss.
One-thing it was not;
Dot became a no-dot.

Dot expanded
Up, down, back, forward, sideways,
For a million billion whatevers
Dot pushed its own envelope
Expanding into the no-nothing
which remained
After no-thing split.

Now no-dot was not-now
And no-dot was not-here;
No-dot had moved somewhere
Between then and there.

It rolled and expanded
At incredible pace
Till not-now became time
And not-here became space.

But no-dot was scattered
Battered and shattered
Finding direction
Was all that now mattered.

Because no-dot was lost
And it looked all around,
No-one to be seen
Not even a sound.

It longed for direction
A place to call home
And it wished that no-thing
Would pick up the phone.

It wished that no-thing
Would drop it a line
Just then no-thing called
'I hope all is fine?'

'Here is your line
It's called "I-me-mine"
Please confine to this line
That leads from up down.'

A line? That was fine
I will slide down this line
That extends from mid-heaven
Into some-body's spine.

In a golden shrine
On top of cloud nine
Line waited its turn,
Line bided its time.

But line became fixed
Compulsive, obsessive
Line would not bend
This got quite excessive.

Dirty or clean
False or be true
There was really no way
To bridge between two.

Two? You said two?
Knock knock! Two of Who?
Two of two, it is us
And we're saying to you –

Line, Look through the keyhole
And see what is new
Break out of your shell
Line, Find the true you.

Set yourself free
I will lend you my strength
Take a step forward
Break out of length

More space to play in
Sheet, surface, square
Combine length and width
There is much power2 there.

You can tilt to the future
Lean back into past
Scratch till it itches
Reach for the stars.

Breadth's what I long for!
Thought line with a sigh
I'm tired of floating
T'ween mud and the sky

I'll have a good stretch
He said with a yawn
I'm bored of this prison
And feeling forlorn

I'm looking to flex
And I'm itching to bend
Time to grow wide now
Time to extend

Tired of this axis
Heaven and earth
I'm taking the plunge
I'm going to give birth!

Line took a step forward
Took a step back
Opened the door
Heard the shell crack

Time twisted and curled
Space was a whirl
Universe dancing
Galaxies swirl

It was time to be long
It was time to be two
And he looked at his mum
And he said 'Hi what's new?

Now a baby's a baby
Until it grows ripe
It functions quite simply
It works like a pipe;

You pump food in one side
Some love and a drink
And it comes out the other
With quite a big stink

It cries and demands
It screams till it gets
It doesn't see others
It doesn't care yet

There's some babies I know
That at age forty two
Can't get satisfaction
And scream till they're blue

So to reach for the stars
Or melt into bliss
They shoot up some junk
Or just take the piss

It's a shallow existence
Of joy, discontent
So we're longing for depth
To give us a vent

As we float in our ark
Side by side, two by two
It's time that we turned
And recognised you.

We'll send out a dove
Open our throat
Find some expression
Get off this old boat

Find us some earth
Let waters recede
Search for a partner
In which to plant seed

To be continued . . .

Space and time

As it moves into a new dimension, Neon loses its orientation in space and time. In addition to the many reports of feeling 'spaced out', the following symptoms illustrate this point.

Three incidences of a miscalculation of where I was in space. I tripped twice going upstairs and once fell over from a standing position on cross-country skis. I don't quite seem to know where my body is in space.

Shortly after taking the remedy, I was confused about where I was.

Heard the sound of my foot move but was not aware of it moving. I did not know where I was.

Neon may also experience a strong sense of disorientation in time.

I had a sense of timelessness and wanted to find the clock but could not. I had no reference points and thought that if I could find out the time, it would be a reference point in the void.

I was confused about my watch. I couldn't tell which way was up on the clock face.

Shortly after waking, I was confused about time, whether it was morning or afternoon.

Moreover, Neon appears to reverse the flow of time:

I remembered incidents in my dreams in reverse order. Very unusual for me

Dreamt she showed me photos of herself getting progressively younger until she was a baby.

The second period, culminating in Neon, initiates the concept of time. One definition of time is attributed to John Wheeler (1911–2008) as follows: *'Time is what prevents everything from happening at once'*[2] or to put it another way, *'Time occurs when now splits'*. At the Hydrogen and Helium levels of unity, time is still one; in the second period this unity splits and begins a backwards and forwards motion.

While there are several references to time in the Neon proving, time is usually considered to have come into being on the fourth day of creation, with the formation appearance of the sun, moon and stars. The heavenly cycles, however, generate circular time rather than linear time, as will become apparent in the study of Krypton. Neon is only a first step into time, the simple division between future and past. (Figure 10.6)

With time pulling in both directions, Neon leans too far into the future, striving towards the new. This may manifest as clairvoyance, an ability to correctly predict future events. It may also manifest as a tendency to rush and hurry. In most cases this is not a pleasant sensation.

Took woman's notes to clinic in case I needed them and she phoned the clinic.

Repeated prophetic notions of daily events before hearing of them, causing anxiety and discomfort: after thinking of a person not seen for months, I found out he had phoned a few days before; depression and sadness unexplained until I heard of sad family news of something that had already happened.

Feel out of control, as if time is moving relentlessly and remorselessly forward and I'm stuck behind, unable to keep up. Panic, guilt, constant anxiety that I won't get it all done.

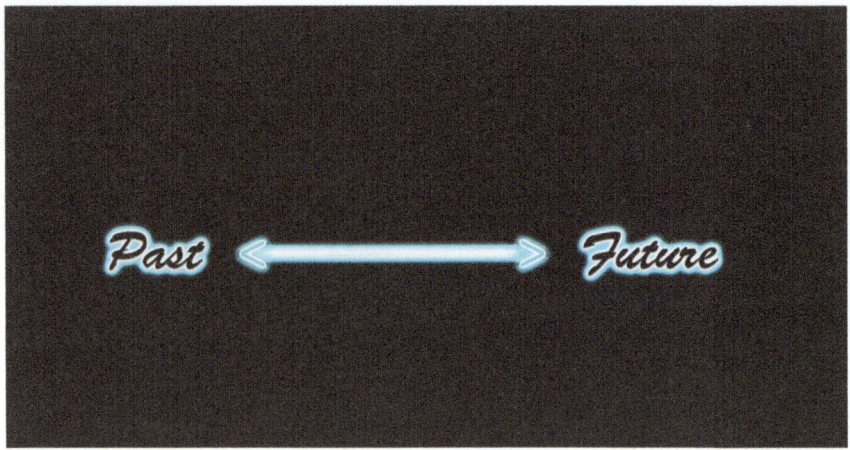

Figure 10.6 *'Now' separates into past and future*

I felt very speedy, and could not get words out fast enough, was tripping over my words.

Impatient with my son, then felt guilty.

Neon may also 'lean' into the past …

Husband comments that I seem 'far away and long ago.' He hasn't seen me this 'gone' in a long time.

For some provers the remedy was curative, bringing them back into the present.

My spirit feels light without being weightless. Prior to taking the remedy, I felt as if I was too far in the future, without realising it. I feel as if I have taken a step back and am in the here and now.

I can't seem to judge time in the past. Can't think back through the days. It's as if I've lost the thread with the past that connects all past days together. It has dissolved. I seem to be more in the moment and less hurried.

References

1   Pascall B. *Pensees* (trans. John Warrington). London: Dent (Everyman's Library No. 874), 1932 Available online at: http://www.stat.ucla.edu/history/pascal_wager.pdf

2   Developer online. Available online at: http://developeronline.blogspot.com/2008/04/time-is-what-keeps-things-happening-all.html

3   Abbott EA. *Flatland: A Romance of Many Dimensions*. Available online at: http://www.geom.uiuc.edu/~banchoff/Flatland/

11

NEON SYNTHESIS

The following is a synthesis of Neon, based on sensations and functions or the 'verb' of the remedy. Please note that sensation and function are interchangeable and form a cycle.[i] They can be read in reverse order so that, for example, *Sensation*: cannot dissolve; *Function*: become fluid can be read as *Sensation*: fluid; *Function*: cannot dissolve.

Synthesis

Sensation: Separated from heaven. Disconnected, stranger, odd one out.
Function: Must unite with the stars.

Sensation: Upright, with direct connection to heaven.
Function: Must divide and lean towards desires.

Sensation: Cannot dissolve.
Function: Become fluid.

Adjectives: Colourful, soluble, blissful, grateful, free, dependent.

Nouns: Water, stars, sky, firmaments, clouds, doors, windows, keyholes, the iris, skin, numbers, reason, lotus, psora, time and space (see Chapter 15).

Image: Oneness opposed by division and separation. Contentment opposing dissatisfaction. Seeking something new breeds desire. The Neon personality may be childish, a two-dimensional personality with lack of emotional depth: I itch, I scratch, I want. Yet if it can transcend the state of a crawling baby and stand upright, Neon may reach contentment and bliss, an effortless energy powered by universal force and mathematical logic. If Neon does not achieve this higher state, life will be a hard, tiring

---

[i] For more information on this method of analysis, see Sherr J. *Dynamic Materia Medica – Syphilis* (2nd edn). Glasgow: Saltire Books, 2014.

and desperate struggle, punctuated by discontent, criticism of self and others and great irritability.

> From Hydrogen's separation from God
> to Neon's split
> we have substituted
> the sun with city lights
> and bliss with discontent.
>
> And the people bowed and prayed
> To the neon god they made.
>   Paul Simon[1]

Chakra: Brow (Pituitary), Sexual (Adrenals)

Day of creation: Second day

Colour: Indigo

Musical scale: A

Whammy: Intellect and physical health.[2]

Location: The oceans, the stars, Atlantis, Las Vegas.

Time: Equinox

Book: *Flatland: A Romance of Many Dimensions.*[3]

Movies: *Pi. The Matrix. Star Wars. Rain Man. Waterworld. ET.*

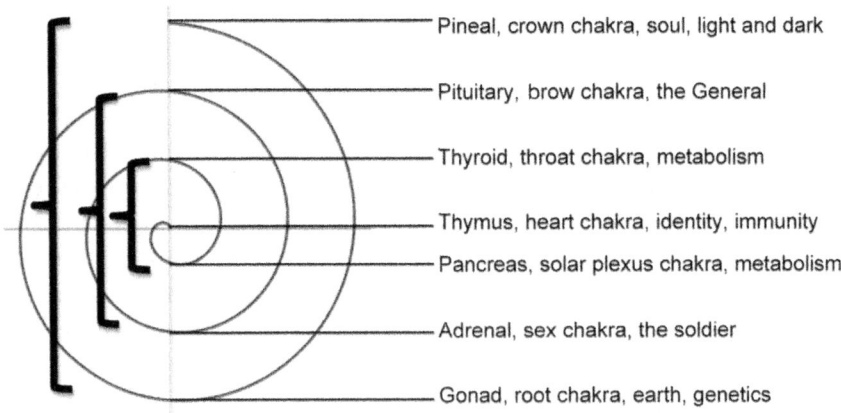

Pineal, crown chakra, soul, light and dark

Pituitary, brow chakra, the General

Thyroid, throat chakra, metabolism

Thymus, heart chakra, identity, immunity

Pancreas, solar plexus chakra, metabolism

Adrenal, sex chakra, the soldier

Gonad, root chakra, earth, genetics

Figure 11.1 Neon relates to the brow chakra of intellect, and to the adrenals of desire

From Shakespeare: Macbeth, Act 2 Scene III[4]

(Knocking within. Enter a Porter.)

Porter:
Here's a knocking indeed! If a
man were porter of hell-gate, he should have
old turning the key.

(Knocking within)

Knock, knock, knock! Who's there, i' the name of
Beelzebub? Here's a farmer, that hanged
himself on the expectation of plenty: come in
time; have napkins enow about you; here
you'll sweat for't.

(Knocking within)

Knock,
knock! Who's there, in the other devil's
name? Faith, here's an equivocator, that could
swear in both the scales against either scale;
who committed treason enough for God's sake,
yet could not equivocate to heaven: O, come
in, equivocator.

(Knocking within)

Knock,
knock, knock! Who's there? Faith, here's an
English tailor come hither, for stealing out of
a French hose: come in, tailor; here you may
roast your goose.

(Knocking within)

Knock,
knock; never at quiet! What are you? But
this place is too cold for hell. I'll devil-porter
it no further: I had thought to have let in
some of all professions that go the primrose
way to the everlasting bonfire.

References

1   Simon P. *The Sound of Silence* (1964). Available online at: http://www.sglyrics.myrmid.com/sounds.htm

2   Seven Whammies: Spirituality, intellect, relationships, occupation, society, sex/wealth/power, home/territory. In: Sherr J. *Dynamic Materia Medica: Helium*. Glasgow: Saltire Books, 2013.

3   Abbott EA. *Flatland. A romance of many dimensions*. Available online at: http://www.math.brown.edu/~banchoff/gc/Flatland/

4   Shakespeare W. Macbeth, Act iii. Scene iii. Available online at: http://www.shakespeare-online.com/plays/mmacbeth_2_3.html

12

NEON CASES

As well as presenting cases from Camilla's, and my own, practices I have collected cases from as many sources as possible to illustrate different aspects of the remedy. I have presented the cases in the form in which they were given to me. Some cases were edited for grammar without changing the meaning.

Some of the follow-ups are long-term and others short. For the purpose of understanding the remedy both are useful. While long-term cures are preferable, I do not subscribe to the notion that one needs years of good follow-ups to learn something about a remedy.

In some situations a remedy may act for a short time with a profound cure; this may indicate a deeper action of the remedy – the susceptibility is fulfilled and that remedy is no longer needed. In other situations the remedy action may be partial. In this case we should note only those symptoms that were cured, as well as any proving symptoms. In acute cases the duration of action is naturally shorter.

CASE 12.1 Acute influenza

Camilla Sherr, Tanzania

Female, age 43

First consultation
'I feel terrible. Bad flu, sinuses, tired and irritable. I have had these symptoms for two weeks and they are not improving.

Bright yellow mucus, glowing, **reminds me of the fluorescent yellow marker pen**. Holding head when blowing nose, < jar.

Headache right temple and right forehead, sharp.

Crackling in ear when blowing nose.

Irritable. Feel put upon, family was over at Christmas, it's like I have a mark on my forehead saying 'please come and walk all over me, I feel used and abused and I'm a fool to let people do it'.

Tired, worse on waking in the morning.

Blowing my nose, sinuses and head full of catarrh, feels like I could blow and blow but still not unblock my nose. There's a lot of mucus and it's coming out but I can't blow enough for it to finish.

I want to tell the truth because it's Christmas, I have to talk plainly with people, I'm always letting things go, it's better to be straight, especially with family members.'

Rx: Neon 200C single dose

Follow-up after three days
'Immediately after the remedy I had to pass stool, I became aware that I was thirsty, became tired, and had the urge to evacuate all evening.

Next day I could feel and think better, could get out of bed, could go to work. Headache was gone. I re-dosed in the afternoon, Felt much better and was good in a meeting. Feeling of being used and abused gone.

Totally better in three days.'

Comment (JS)
The main indication for Neon in this case was the fluorescent nasal discharge that also appears in the proving. This was my own proving symptom, the only significant one I had and I was proud of it. I still remember waking up in the middle of the night, blowing my nose and seeing the glowing discharge. I was astounded and tried to show

my wife, who was not amused. I was later even more surprised to find that my supervisor had recorded the symptom as: 'Delusion he has glowing mucus'. I feel redeemed by this case.

Other pointers were the dissatisfaction, the feeling of being abused, the irritability and the need to speak the plain truth, which are common to the noble gases. The need to talk 'straight' fits the Neon verb. The comment about a mark on the forehead is interesting given the location of the headache and Neon's relationship to the brow chakra.

CASE 12.2 Water works

Camilla Sherr, Tanzania

Female, age 44

First consultation
Observation: A very childish woman.

She says repeatedly: 'It is my water works, it's all about my water works' (meaning urinary system). She has had these problems for many years, allopathy has not helped.

She has oedema – watery swellings in her whole body, legs, arms, fingers and ankles.

Her urination is scanty.

She is like a little girl in her marriage; she speaks about her husband and marriage in a childish way, like a little girl. Very naïve.

She is anti-social and not interested in company. She has no contact with her husband and feels separate in the relationship.

It is difficult to get much information out of her. She keeps repeating in a childish voice: 'It's just my water works you know'. 'I feel like I'm dissolving'.

Rx: Neon 200C

Follow-up two months later
All swelling and urinary problems are much better.

Marriage much better, the connection with her husband is much improved. She is much more social. Appears more grown up.

Rx: None

Improvement continued for a year on the one dose, not seen since.

Comment (JS)
This case is quite straight forward. The patient's naïve personality is two dimensional, She repeats the same naïve idiom in a very childish way. The emphasis on 'water' in the way she describes her urinary problems, plus her sense of disconnection and aversion to company, are all indications of Neon. Her sensation of dissolving, which is the exact language of the proving, clinches the choice of remedy.

CASE 12.3 Moonstone

Jeremy Sherr, Tanzania

Female, age 51

First consultation
Observation: her voice is hoarse and indistinct.

She is a retired teacher, but found her work very stressful. She has had homoeopathy in past. Phosphorus helped initially, the best six months of her life, 'I was moon walking', but then she went to higher potencies and it aggravated. Since then she has been oversensitive to remedies. She has had a lot more Phosphorus, but it didn't help.

She also had Sepia, Pulsatilla and Ferrum phosphoricum.

Observation: Speech is unclear.

'Everything affects my eyes. Sensitive to strip lights and neon lights, which aggravate.

High blood pressure, 190/120, always had it. I think I had a minor stroke. My voice is very slurred.

Too much saliva and sinuses are congested.

I was adopted. My real mother killed herself. [*Observation:* She is crying. She continues to cry through most of the interview.] Adopted at very early age, don't know my father. This is heavy. I was raised in a violent family. [Crying.] My adoptive mother married a vicious, alcohol-dependent man. I protected her from age 11. He was vicious and raging. [She is crying all the time.] I wanted to protect my adoptive mother. I was sad and angry. I stood up to him always, I wasn't scared. Rage and sadness because of what he was doing to my mother. He tried to get into bed with me.

Very hoarse throat. I can't articulate words properly, people can't understand me. Sad about my voice, I had a good strong voice before.

Very strong carotid pulse.

Saliva, profuse morning.

I am an oversensitive person, very reactive. I worry myself into a state, put a hex on myself. Much better if reassured. I put others before myself.

Many illnesses throughout my life.

I don't need to be needed, don't need to look after a lot of people. My marriage broke apart, I felt devastated, abandoned, like at the beginning of my life. But I enjoy life, friends and have a good time [she says while crying].

Before Phosphorus I used to struggle with depression in the morning, I had morning low fever > Phosphorus.

I have many pedunculated and cauliflower warts.

I am vegan, love animals. I don't smoke or drink, I do yoga.

I lost my voice after many friends had cancer, it took a lot out of me.

Suicidal after marriage broke up. I attempted suicide at 31, was saved. I feel despair, abandoned. I'm not depressed [repeats many times]. Usually I am very positive.

Cared for parents for 20 years. My adoptive mother said, 'You have bad blood, no one wanted you'. As a child I didn't love her, but had to protect her. [She continues to cry all the time.] My greatest sadness was when my real mother killed herself. I was 12 at the time but didn't find out till I was 13. [Crying.] I stood up to my stepfather. I was courageous, he was vicious. Stood up to him, knocked him out. Mother closed down, I went into overdrive.

Fear of dark and thunderstorms in past but now that is better. I used to see ghosts. Sensitive to atmosphere, ghosts, dark.

Menorrhagia during menopause.

Aversion to heat and cold, extremes.

Dreams of angels, I love angels. I like images of angel wings protecting me and enfolding me. I love stained glass and light reflected on water. I have dreams of moonstones. I love the stars. I am an airy Gemini. I like to look at the moon, it's calming. I like glitter and luminosity.

I used to have a lot of self-loathing but I now love myself. I avoid relationships for fear of being abandoned, but I am brave enough to travel alone, do things alone.'

Rx: Neon 30C single dose

Follow-up 6 weeks later
'Much better. I feel much calmer. I can't feel my blood rushing around like before. Much calmer and stronger. No anxiety at all. I am much, much happier. Taking things in my stride again.

Within 4 four hours of taking the remedy, my jaw was looser and I could talk better. Articulation has improved a lot. My voice is more consistent.

Much more energy and motivation. I had no aggravation on the remedy. My eyes did not look exhausted as they have after other remedies in the past.

My boundaries feel better.

Dream: I was consoling the devil in his loneliness. He was disguised as an old woman. I was not afraid of him. He was a fallen angel. I love angels.

I am so happy!'

Rx: Neon 30C in two weeks time

Follow-up 2 months later
'Feeling very well, lighter, more fluid in my body.

My voice is much stronger and clearer. Breathing is much better. The saliva is much less. Sinuses are much better.

I feel very positive, energy is fine, I am coping with life very well. I am less haunted by the past and family.

Pulse has slowed down. Blood pressure lower. Much calmer. No crying, no sadness, just positive. I had a very positive dream about work, I was getting very good feedback at work. I heard someone calling my name in my dreams. Very good dreams.'

Rx: Neon 30C when needed. (In case of relapse)

Follow-up three months later
She repeated Neon once.

'Doing very well, Neon has really helped me. Much calmer, more productive. I am working on my house. No anxiety, feeling lighter and brighter, managing life better and feeling positive.

My blood pressure remains high, but it has been like that all my life and I don't expect it to change. However, I take no medication and feel OK. No more headaches and no more dizziness.

Voice is becoming more articulate, people understand me better.

I exercise more, put myself first more often, feel strong and not weepy.

Dreamt of a serene, inspiring Japanese woman, felt drawn to her. Can't get a song out of my head '*The Greatest Love*' by Barbra Streisand. I am opening up to the possibility of needing someone! I feel much stronger, Neon has done me a lot of good, I'm coping so well, no more despair, so happy that I want to dance.'

Rx: Neon 30C when needed

Comment (JS)
My assessment is that this lady was in a state of severe depression. I chose Neon because of the aggravation from neon lights, the attraction to the moon, stars and angels, light and luminosity, as well as the strong contradiction between happiness and optimism on the one hand, and deep despair on the other. Her general demeanour was childish and naïve.

CASE 12.4 Ice boy

Jeremy Sherr, Tanzania

Male, age 2½

First consultation

The boy has previously taken Lycopodium, Tuberculinum bovinum, Phosphorus, Veratrum album, Staphysagria and Medorrhinum with no results.

Completely obsessed with opening and closing doors. If a door is open, he has to close it. If it's closed, he'll open and close it, open and close it, open and close it. This is driving everyone crazy. If the lid of the rubbish bin is open, he has to close it. If a drawer is open, he closes it.

Afraid of dogs, has been all his life. He will climb as high as he can on his pram to avoid them.

Craves ice, ice cream and salt. When his mother was pregnant with him she had a huge craving for ice. The little boy will sit happily in a restaurant as long as he has a glass full of ice and is free to munch away on it. He will go to the freezer and help himself to ice cream. He could live off it.

Another huge craving is for salt. When walking in a mall, he'll grab the salt from a café table and eat straight from it.

He is destructive. If he sees a pile of magazines or books on the table he will push them onto the floor. Does not like piles. He throws things, anything, all the time. On the other hand, he is noticeably nonviolent and never hits. He gives away all his toys willingly and doesn't stand up for himself. He is very kind, gentle and caring.

He very much likes to play by himself. If there are other children around he will take his books and go to another room to read. He is very self-contained, almost to a fault. He observes everything but doesn't really communicate that much.

His mother read an article about autism and became intensely worried since her boy displayed an alarming number of the symptoms. However there was no diagnosis.

His favourite words are 'clouds', 'sun', 'sky' and 'moon.' He keeps repeating these. He loves to gaze at the clouds.

He loves water, baths and beaches with big waves. He was born in the water and has a Grand Trine in water astrologically.

Constantly brushes his nose, as if it's itchy.

He loves to spy on people.

He is obsessed with the number ten. He will count to ten in three languages and always pauses dramatically before he gets to ten – and then everybody has to clap and cheer.

His all-time favourite story is the one where Winnie the Pooh goes knocking on all his friends' doors, but finds that nobody is home.

The astrologer says he will be a great spiritual teacher when he is older.

Rx: Neon 200C

Follow-up
Immediately calmed down and stopped throwing things.

When his mother offered him ice cubes he just looked at them and said 'They're cold.' He stopped asking for ice cream and stopped eating salt completely.

These were dramatic changes in light of the fact that none of the previous remedies had ever made a difference. His language took a giant leap forward and he started communicating in a way he had never been able to before. And his obsession with doors ended, much to everyone's relief!

Two days after the remedy he wanted to walk the neighbour's dog on the leash!

He suddenly grew a lot and changed from a baby to a little boy almost overnight. He interacts much more now with other children.

He also stopped rubbing his nose.

He continued to do well for many months, and Neon has remained a good remedy for him.

Comment (JS)
The obvious clues were the opening and closing of doors, the desire to spy and the obsession with numbers, especially the number ten, as well as water, clouds and sky. His self-contained, gentle disposition and childish behaviour confirmed the remedy. While cravings for ice and salt are not mentioned in the proving, they are both related to water. Anecdotal clues are the fixation with Winnie the Pooh, knocking on doors, and the 'future as a spiritual teacher'. At the time I did not understand the aversion to three-dimensional 'piles',

wanting everything level on the floor; but it reveals that he is stuck in the second dimension, that of surfaces, doors and windows. Clinical additions are 'Fear of dogs, desire for ice and nose, rubbing'.

CASE 12.5 HIV/AIDS

Camilla Sherr, Tanzania

Female, age unknown

First consultation
She was diagnosed as HIV positive in 2004 and has been on antiretro-viral medications (ARVs) since 2008. Since taking ARVs, her CD4 count has risen from 112 to 189, which was her last count a week ago, March, 2009.

She is very worried about how to raise her children. None of her kids is HIV positive.

She has itching of the skin, scars on her legs and the beginnings of Kaposi's sarcoma.

She experiences headaches, with pulsing pain in her temples, worse when she thinks about being unemployed and worries where she will find money to feed the family. She's worried about getting pregnant and wants to have her tubes tied.

She has severe pain in the chest when breathing.

Before taking ARVs, she had a dream that her mother passed away and she woke up crying. She also had a dream that someone was knocking on the door, but when she went to open it no one was there.

She likes being with people and cracking jokes, making people laugh.

She has a very poor appetite and is losing weight. She also suffers from nausea. Generally she feels weak and it is difficult for her to walk or work.

She is thirsty.

When she was diagnosed, she took the news positively. Her husband rejected her after the test and told her to leave. She was very hurt. Now she has to survive alone and she worries about the children.

Rx: Neon 30C Double dose

Follow-up one month later
Headache and chest pains are gone. No more nausea. Appetite better. Itching is mostly gone.

She has no more weakness. She says she is doing fantastically on the remedy and feels strong and happy.

Rx: None

Follow-up five months later
'I just came to say I feel so well! The nausea and all my other symptoms are gone. I'm feeling strong and I have a very good appetite! I can work, so the money problems are not as bad.'

Rx: Neon 12C daily

Follow-up six months later
'I haven't been to see you since October because I have been feeling so well. Everything has been OK and my symptoms are gone. The remedy finished three months ago. But in the last few weeks I've had a cough.'

The cough is worse from motion.

Rx: Bryonia alba 30C three times daily

Follow-up two days later
Cough is gone, feeling better.

Rx: Resume Neon 12C daily

Comment (JS)
This is a typical African HIV/AIDS case. There are a very few general symptoms, no useful modalities, and very few individualising mental symptoms (the money worries and anxiety about how to bring up the kids are very common in Africa). The clue came from one of the dreams. Dreams are often the 'strange rare and peculiar' of African patients, the other side that can express the idiosyncrasy freely. It is common for us to rely on one significant dream, because there is little

else, and it works well. In this instance the dream of someone 'knocking on the door but finding no one there' is straight out of the Neon proving. Combine this with the positive attitude and cheerful personality and you have a prescription. While this might seem two dimensional, the dream world is the window to the next dimension. I would not say that Neon is high on the list of pandemic remedies for HIV/AIDS in Africa, but we have used it a few times, as opposed to the other nobles, which we have never used in this context.

CASE 12.6 Preaching from the rooftops

Jeremy Sherr, Tanzania

Male, age unknown

First consultation
Diagnosed HIV positive, April 2010. Began antiretroviral treatment (ARVs) at the same time. CD4 was then 136, now down to 98. This indicates that the ARV medication has stopped working.

Pain and swelling in both legs.

He had diarrhoea before ARVs. Now, only occasionally.

Main complaint is that he feels extremely weak, especially while walking. Finds it difficult to do physical work or walk long distances. His legs feel heavy. No work means no money to feed his family.

Pain in forehead.

Vision is poor.

Some vertigo.

Tongue pale with white coating.

Frequent urine, which can be very scanty.

Profuse perspiration at night.

Appetite poor.

Numbness legs and fingers. Occasional swelling of legs.

Sleep poor.

His wife ran away but he doesn't mind.

Dream that he is flying and lands on the roof tops and is blessing people from there. In the dream he can bless people, but when wakes he feels alone.

He is happy. He says nothing bothers him other than having no work.

Rx: Neon 200C twice a week for a month

Follow-up six weeks later
'Thank you very much, the remedy helped a lot! I feel much better.'

Now he is stronger and can walk long distances. The heaviness in the legs is much better, the swelling is almost gone. His energy is much better now, he can farm and work. Before he had to lie down often.

Headache is better.

He feels like he is cured.

Appetite is better, he eats much more. Before he had no appetite and at times would go two days without eating.

Vertigo is gone.

Vision is much better, can even read now.

Urine is normal now, not frequent or scanty.

Perspiration at night has stopped.

No more numbness in extremities.

Sleep is much better. No dreams.

He feels much better in himself, strong and healthy.

Rx: Neon 200C once a week

Follow-up three months later
He is totally well. The remedy helped a lot.

Legs are much better, no pain or swelling, he is eating well and feels strong.

All other symptoms are much better. 'There is no problem'.

No CD4 check yet.

Rx: Neon 12C daily (I did not have any 200C)

Six months after starting the remedy he came to see me, dressed in a suit (highly unusual in Africa). He dressed up specially to thank me. He feels very well and strong all round and is working and making money.

Comment (JS)
This is another case of HIV/AIDS in Africa. The patient was very bubbly and cheerful. Water issues feature strongly in the case: Frequent and scanty urination, perspiration, diarrhoea and swelling. His dream of blessing people from the rooftops is typical of the 'spiritual teacher' aspect of Neon, as are his happiness and lack of concern about his adverse circumstances (disease, wife leaving him). From the Neon proving we have – *Dream of being a successful spiritual teacher. Dream of being in a crowd with a spiritual teacher.*

It is interesting that the patient's main concern was his weakness while walking, but after the remedy he was very excited about his ability to walk long distances with ease, a prominent feature of the Neon proving.

CASE 12.7 'I have arrived in the sphere of the earth'

Maria Schmelzer-Schenkel, Bochum, Germany[i]

Acknowledgments: I want to thank my Aikido friend Chris Lang for his great help translating this article into English.

Female, age 40

First consultation March 8th, 2004
She suffers from exhaustion since pneumonia in January, 2004.

The case history: Panic attacks since 2002. In recent years recurrent sinusitis and bronchitis during the winter. Headaches for many years. Joint pains recurring since the age of 18. Nausea and stomach pain since childhood. Operation for a paralytic ileus with staphylococcal sepsis at age 18, before her final school exams.

She has been given many remedies with all kingdoms represented: Staph, Calc-c, Lyc, Cupr, Sep, Nat-m, Plat, Nux-v, Sil.

Her symptoms have improved slowly on these remedies; however, there has been no change in her overall condition. Mrs. X experiences these times as severe, disabling and distressing.

The following themes emerge repeatedly, alone or accompanied by various physical ailments:

---

[i] For a longer version of this article see: Schlingensiepen-Brysch I. Sprechende Quellen – Eine Schöpfung entfaltet sich. *Systematische Homöopathie, Band 2.*

Fears: that everything is uncontrollable; of being seriously ill; that she doesn't have long to live. Fear of dying: 'I feel the limitations of time.' Frequent dreams that she will die. Feels threatened. Perceives threats in the room, often all night long. Wakes with a start at night, sees dark figures, animals, or devils. Must turn on the light. Patient: 'I want to seek safety, but cannot. Fear of going insane.'

Questioning what life is all about. Existential anxiety: about being destroyed, extinguished. Feels she has no home, feels forlorn, lonely and disrupted. Angry: 'parents didn't give a fuck about me.' Powerless, 'lashing about me.' Rage: 'I want to liberate myself but I don't get through. A huge tidal wave washes me away; I'm sinking, I'm losing myself.'

'Everything is leaving upwards. Lightness, as if something were moving upwards. An elevated feeling: I feel only my head and nothing below. I can't feel myself, can't be inside myself. No control, unable to do anything. Sensation of having no fundament. Fundament represents security, being here.'

I undertake the first steps of the Source Method with the patient.

During this time, Mrs. X is in a state of deep crisis.

Follow-up February 3rd, 2006

Patient: 'My father died of lung cancer. It was a stressful time.'

Doctor: 'How did you experience the death of your father?/Patient: 'Like a shock. Suddenly he was no longer there. Then I was very busy, there were thousands of things to take care of.

Sudden fear that I would have an allergic reaction while eating. That I would have convulsions or suddenly collapse, be cut off and gone'.

Doctor: 'Is there any bodily sensation when these feelings arise?'

At this point the patient descends into her inner world. She speaks very slowly, often breaks off, her vision is directed inwards.

Patient: 'I feel I am mainly in my head. My head feels heavy, the rest is transparent, an empty shell. A "nothing" feeling. As if I was not here. As if I were emotionally cut off, as if I could no longer perceive myself. Not as matter: unable to hold, to sense, to feel. As if my body did not belong to me. A mass. Dissolving. A vibration within. Like gas wafting around. Like tubes, wafting, vibrating, oscillating.'

Doctor: 'What is the opposite of that?'

Patient: 'Being hard, holding, being here.' [Gesture: The patient grabs her arm tightly.]

Doctor: 'And the opposite of that?'

Patient: 'Being permeable, being penetrated. Emptiness. Cut off. I know that there is something, but cannot feel it. Transparent, like a foil, clear sight. Waves, sinus curve. A foil like a shell, pores, where anything can enter. Where there is a gas, compressed energy. Big bang, primordial soup. Honeycomb-like, absorbing, imbibing. Penetrating through pores, swallowing everything, it dissolves. Sulphur, cesspool, where everything rots. The material dissolves. Decay, decomposition, fumes. End of the material. Gas rises. Mercury, foil-like. Something that doesn't hold, something with no real metallic properties. In another world, not here on earth. Not really here, cut off. Energies that I can tap into.'

I pick up on one of the many terms which Mrs. X has used. I choose a word which should not lead her too much.

Doctor: 'Describe "dissolve".'

Patient: 'My body feels like a gas. It feels as if particles are drifting apart and floating away. Nothing is holding, things are not slotting together any more. Everything falls apart, body awareness slips away. A sensation of being pulled apart. Particles, bubbles are pulled apart and disperse as if they can no longer hold actively together, as if acted upon by a kind of suction. Different forces, such as large magnets, are at work, pulling in different directions. A completely empty space. All slides apart because nothing can hold together. The binding forces are missing. I am pulled up, I rise upwards. The feeling is most noticeable in my feet. A feeling of being transparent, of having no hold. There is no identity, it is something neutral, something that can't be touched. A paradox, it evaporates, it is defenceless; nothing and nobody can grab it. Everything passes through. Even male-female is gone, a neutral feeling.

If one wakes up, one doesn't know where one is. One misjudges things, takes things from a dream. Presence in space, chaos, diffusion. There are forward-looking dreams. Like a spaceman. Like carbonated bubbles.'

Doctor: 'Is there anything in nature which is exactly like this?'

But nothing came to her mind – **that's what she says!!!**

And so, my thoughts are wandering around:

Somehow she has described this thing clearly, precisely and with great intensity, but what might it be? The question about the physical sensation brought up so much. Why wasn't she able to identify the substance?

I thought it was probably something from the periodic table, she gave so many physical terms. The theme was existence: the second row. But the tube, what might that be?

I noted possible remedies. Amongst them was the 'source remedy', but also some drug remedies.

In the aftermath she describes again: 'Not complete anymore, like a shell. Like a small, contracted point. Crystal, freezing, being petrified. Being destroyed, that hurts overall. As if breaking into pieces. Like lightning, which passes through. A ball of fire inside, burning and scorching everything. A tearing, a division into four parts.

Fear of being isolated, of being abandoned. Vacuum. Only emptiness and floating. Falling and nothing to hold on. Like an astronaut floating in space.

The 'I' is not there. The positive side is that I am not available. It is a shelter, a vacuum, no one gets through, it is a safety zone. Like a big empty house. Take cover, seek shelter. As if the senses are paralyzed, you are absolutely unable to react. It feels like being in a movie. As if the intellect had been there all those years and had left the emotions behind. Anxiety, loneliness, at somebody's mercy, shock, paralysis. Everything is focused on my eyes. They feel large and there is pressure. I have to stay in control. My existence is somehow threatened. The vital force breaks away. The mood breaks away.'

In September, 2006, the patient had an MRI of her cervical spine because of pain in her left arm. A herniated disc was diagnosed.

Follow-up November 14th, 2006
'My left arm is a bit better since Feldenkrais therapy, but there's a strange feeling of powerlessness in my arm with heat and nausea. I have another stye on my left eye. A dry feeling like sand paper on my upper eyelid and pain shooting into the eye, stitching like a needle.

All this relates to my mood: to my search for the ultimate. I have always done a lot of reading. Again and again the question arises: What holds the world together at its interior? None of the answers endure. The internal debate continues. There is peace when I feel connected, but then the reason, the intellect questions: This is not enough, this cannot endure, what is the sense, the origin? Where am I?

You have to accept that there are no answers. It is a feeling of being lifted off. The answer is maybe to be more present, to discuss less. It was as if I had become immaterial, something not of the flesh. As if the spiritual part, the eternal part were connected to the other world, while one foot remained in this one. As if I were a character in a movie, but did not play the character myself. As if I had left my body and were hovering above it.

A connection to the primordial ground.

Rx: Neon 200C

I did not tell the patient the name of the remedy.

I still remember the conversation in which she so vividly described her bodily sensations, and hope that she will be able to go all the way to the source. Later it became clear that Mrs. X had long since gone all the way to the source, though silently.

Follow-up January 17th, 2007
'That evening after taking the remedy, I was standing at the window, looking outside and thinking "I have stopped here now, I have arrived in the sphere of the earth."

The daily diarrhoea after breakfast suddenly stopped. But I have had stomach complaints similar to those I had as a child. I had such terrible constipation when I was little that my bowels had to be cleared manually. I just did not want to go to the toilet. The scar from the ileus operation (1982) has been hurting.

Emotionally, I am explosive and have been reacting physically. I got into a physical fight with my mother. These feelings have never before been so severe or lasted so long. My threshold is low, the barrier is thin, I quickly react physically. I need to maintain better boundaries, then I would not be so absorbed by everything and would feel more stable.

The fear has been farther away. I used to fantasise about disasters and about being seriously ill, with fear of death. I've been waking up every night with anxiety from a dream. In the dream I am already 60 years old. I wonder might it feel like this when you are dying? Panic about dying. As if frozen, I somehow do exist, but cannot do anything. As if the rigour persisted. I hover about unable to do anything. Darkness, but more "I" in the dream. I have never before had a feeling of "I" or a sense of existence during the day. Now it is there in my dreams.

My menses have been troublesome. I have pain in my left arm.'

Rx: Wait

At the end of the follow up on April 20th, 2007, I told the patient the remedy. A big surprise was in store not only for me but also for Mrs. X:

Patient: 'Do you remember when I was talking about a tube? Didn't I refer to a 'neon tube'? I didn't say it out loud, but the words came to my mind.'

Doctor: 'Please describe what you were thinking at that time.'

Patient: 'The neon tube, so fragile and translucent. Outside only a very thin, brittle glass and inside a wafting.'

Rx: Wait (Neon 200C to hold)

Follow-up May 13th, 2011

The patient comes for treatment again after a break of about a year.

Patient: 'Mentally I feel good. I have a new love. But certain physical things are coming up again in waves. Dizziness and headaches every month, related to my periods. For about one and a half years I've had the feeling that I'm in menopause. Actually, I do not feel so old. I experience this as something positive. It helps me to slow down at work. I'm more aware that existence is finite. Irritable bladder: I have the urge to go, but not a lot happens. I had this problem 15 or 20 years ago. It's been back again in the last year and a half.

Violent restlessness in my left leg, an unpleasant tension in the ankle. It's an old symptom, back again in the last year and a half. What is different now is the spasms – my leg shoots up. I've been having muscle spasms all over – on my buttocks, legs, back, arms, and corners of my mouth. Shallow, tense breathing with the restlessness. A paradoxical breathing, instead of going down to the diaphragm, I draw it up.

Twitching helps to relieve the tension, exercise helps me to relax. I am involved in so many things. I am aware that I should extract myself from the stressful process and slow down. When I do that, my neck pain lessens. It helps with "existence". I have headaches with nausea and sensitivity to light, mostly on the left side. They start in my neck and extend towards my face. Sometimes they are pulsating, sometimes there is a strong pulling sensation. They make me dizzy and affect my concentration.

I can deal better with all complaints, as I feel better psychologically. My belly is much better. However, dizziness in bed at night is new. As if the bed were moving, it's like being on a ship. I am spinning in the same direction as the bed. As if the ground were shaking, turning like a carousel and I were moving with it. It knocks me to the side.

Many dreams of being in company, making plans to go out and have a drink. I am looking forward to it. Dream: I'm going down a mountain thinking "this is crazy, you with your vertigo, you will never get back." Then I sit astride a rock, as if on a horse and I'm frozen because of my fear of heights. I shout and people in the valley below hear me. Next thing, I am down in the valley and see a woman on the rock. She is saved by 5 or 6 people. It is a good feeling of trust. I am sure they will come. What is new is that I ask for help, I am no longer the lonesome fighter. Previously, autonomy was the highest commandment.

I have more physical symptoms, so I feel my body but psychologically I feel good.'

Rx: Neon 1M

Follow-up June, 2011, three weeks after taking Neon 1M
Her physical symptoms are not better. The restlessness and tension are worse and this aggravates her exhaustion.

Rx: Neon 50M

As soon as she held the remedy in her hand, Mrs. X said 'I feel calmer.'

Follow-up August 5th, 2011
'Emotionally and physically I feel good. The headaches during my menses were milder and bladder complaints are gone. The restlessness and twitching have definitely improved. I'm more balanced. I still get slight dizziness from time to time, but only for a few moments. I still

have dreams of being in company and anxious dreams. I call out and someone comes to help me.'

Comment (JS)

This case, sent by Maria, is based on the Source method, in which the patient will at some point describe, or even name, the remedy they need. There are many references in the case to a gas-like state, which I have combined into one paragraph below:

Like gas wafting around; the feeling of lightness and being elevated, permeable, evaporates, transparent, emptiness, floating, gas rises. No real metallic properties. My body feels like a gas. Bubbles are pulled apart and disperse. Like a spaceman.

And finally, the source appears: *The neon tube, so fragile and translucent. Outside only a very thin, brittle glass and inside a wafting.*

The noble gas theme of being 'emotionally cut off' is clearly perceptible. The most essential part of the case, however, is a lack of connection to the earth, a sensation of there being no 'I': *'What is the sense, the origin? Where am I?'*

This state is echoed by the *'Sensation of having no fundament'*, *'a feeling of being lifted off, as if one foot is in the eternal world, while one foot remained in this one'*. This hovering between two worlds makes it difficult to differentiate between Helium and Neon. But in addition to the source description, the following themes point us in the direction of Neon. There is an affinity to water, such as *'A huge tidal wave washes me away'; 'I'm sinking'*, and, most importantly, the mention of *'dissolving'* three times in the case, a prominent Neon word. There is a lack of any sense of 'I', like a baby who has not yet separated from his mother. This is somewhat reflected in this watery image: *Vertigo as like being on a ship.*

Following the remedy she develops a stronger sense of self identity. There is a slow landing on earth, which echoes the language of the proving perfectly. The patient says: *I have arrived in the sphere of the earth*. While the proving states: At last, I touch the earth.

CASE 12.8 Holding on, letting go

Mary Aspinwall, USA

Female, age 28

First consultation
Lives with her partner and their son, age 3.

Main complaint: Abnormal menstrual bleeding.

'I bleed heavily for 17–21 days of the month with spotting at other times. Occasional floods of blood with clots the size of prunes. I use 2–3 cloth pads together and have to change them hourly.'

Diagnosis: Fibroid

'I'm tired, depleted, drained and hungry. The hunger is made worse because I'm still breast-feeding. I'm anxious about weaning my son.'

Son's birth: Born at home. Placenta was retained. She lost two-thirds of her blood volume. On the way to the hospital she was separated from her husband and son and told she may die. The placenta had to be manually removed, which was extremely traumatic and painful. She couldn't speak or move after the blood loss and it took a long time for her strength to return. She had an emergency blood transfusion that helped her.

Patient's report: 'I'm very close to my son. He needs me a lot. He hangs on to me. I'm always nervous with a lot on my mind. Being a mother is a responsibility. I am released less often, time for myself is harder to come by. I want to get out without the family. I hold on to the pride of being a good mother and wife, but it's a burden. I never catch up on sleep. It's hard to be calm and let go and do things for myself.

It's hard for me to let go completely. When I had the haemorrhage (after his birth) I couldn't hold on to him. I wanted to make it up to him. I wanted to prove to him I wasn't going to leave him. I felt guilty – I had this ideal, I wanted to cocoon him. I am afraid to release too much. I want to edit everything that comes into my son's life. If I were to release and let go, everything would fall apart. I want him to be secure – I'm going to hold on to him. Something could happen to my son when he is with my husband. Kids die from things you don't expect. I can see him choking or falling.'

Relationship with partner: 'He is very cerebral, it causes me a lot of stress. I want him to enter our world (hers and her son's).

Contentment. . . . It is wonderful, it is everything I wanted. I wanted to be a mother, a housewife. This is the place I am supposed to be.'

Analysis
Holding on/releasing or letting go.

The sensation is: if I don't hold on, everything will fall apart. Releasing is dangerous – she holds on to the placenta and when it is forcibly taken, her body releases too much blood. She has to hold on to life, for her son's sake. Now she wants to hold on to him, but still she is not safe and her body is releasing too much blood, leaving her weak and unable to hold on to him (she has to wean him).

Homoeopath: 'Tell me more about holding on. More about releasing.'

Client: 'Holding on, like the Virgin Mary. Very dark greens and shimmery blacks, darker in the middle. A tunnel. Anxiety. A void. Space. A very cold colour/foreign.

As if you could get pulled into it. A force, very strong, sucking and pulling, but the body relaxes. Fear and confusion, but calming. Vibrating. Buzzing. Electrical.

The nurse told me I needed to calm down because I was dying (weeps). I was between two worlds. I heard whispery, female, fairy voices. I realised there was a possibility that my son could grow up without me and I had to be there for him. I never thought about me. When he was in my body I had felt better than I ever felt before. He needed me.'

Sankaran's schema: Neon – I am separate and content with separation.

Holding separation/birth/I just need one thing to exist, loss of existence, existence threatened by death, fear of losing/separation more than is necessary.

Like being in transition in labour–the space between the dilation phase and the pushing phase. It felt like a big letting go.

Follow-up
Very good remedy reaction: large fibroid gone within a month. All other symptoms also much better. Six months later she was very well with normal menses and much less anxiety around her son.

Much later I received this e-mail:

'I had to write to you because you've been in my thoughts lately. As you probably know already, I'm about to have my second baby. We're so excited. I don't know if you remember my history, but my first son's birth ended up being a pretty dramatic event. After a few years, I ended up with a tumor in my uterus that you treated me for. Your treatment was instrumental in my overall recovery from both the tumor and the lingering effects of the trauma of my son's birth. Unfortunately, the tumor (*fibroid*) was just too big and I did end up with surgery to remove it. *(I did not know it had returned or of course I would have suggested retaking Neon – Mary)*

When I found out I was pregnant, I expected to feel the stress of remembering my son's birth, but to my surprise, as I played it over and over in my head, I realised that I am truly healed. My thoughts kept going back to sitting in your office, the connections you were able to make and the remedy I received. I realised that through this therapy, I was able to somehow put all of that anxiety into my tumor. When it was removed, a veil was lifted and I'm so pleased to say that I'm going into this birth with complete confidence. So, I wanted to make sure that you know how much I appreciate your true gift and how it still plays an important role in my current situation.

Thank you Thank you Thank you Mary.'

Her subsequent delivery went well – Mary

Comment (JS)

Mary has used Sankaran's schema of 'Contented with separation' that is opposed by 'Fear of losing her existence'.

The main susceptibility of the case is the mother-child connection, its epicentre at the moment just before birth, which is precisely the Neon point of stuckness; the point of bursting out of the cocoon to new life, or as the mother put it, 'between two worlds'. As Mary indicates, this manifests in the tension between holding on and letting go.

Added to this are Neon's sense of contentment and its opposing guilt. The Neon proving also has the heavy menses, with clots, that feature in the case.

It is interesting to note the following proving symptom in regards to this case: Like being in transition in labour–the space between the dilation phase and the pushing phase. It felt like a big letting go.

CASE 12.9 Odd one, likes even

Geoff Johnson, UK

Male, age 3

First consultation
Blonde, slight build. Comes into clinic, goes to toybox and starts playing – no interaction.

In last two months he has refused to have a bath – screams and throws things, yet loves standing under sprinkler on lawn. Won't eat anything away from home. Shy, averse unfamiliar food. Only eats pasta, baked beans, biscuits and mushrooms – very definite about this.

Won't join in party games, doesn't bother with other kids unless playing with the toy he likes. However, he is kind and wheels smaller boys around in his tractor. He is happy with his own company and will play by himself for 40 minutes. If bullied, he walks away. He doesn't retaliate and doesn't get upset.

He knows his mind and makes it up firmly. He is fascinated by the number two: his mum was a twin and only played with her sister. He likes his toys in even numbers. Fabulous at jigsaws.

Physically advanced and climbs well – great balance. Speech – slightly behind.

Wakes grouchy. Likes routine – he will say 'It's time for the shower now mummy'.

Tends to constipation.

Very sympathetic. Was upset to see an old man suffering. He kept giving him tissues and wouldn't leave the room.

Rx: Neon 200C twice a day for two days

Follow-up two months later
Overall, a very good improvement, his mother is happy. Mixes well and interacts much more with other children. He will eat a much wider range of food.

Rx: Wait

Patient continued to improve for many months afterwards.

Comment (JS)
Obviously, the main indication for Neon in this case is the obsession with the number two and even numbers. This evenness may be an aspect of his talent for balancing. Add to that the water issues: aversion to bathing and love of sprinklers, aversion to company and the need for routine, and Neon becomes the prescription of choice.

CASE 12.10 Ten-year cycles

Hazel Rank-Broadley, UK

Female, age 57

First consultation May 25, 2007
Main complaint: 'The miseries of an over-active thyroid'.

P. 'Another 10-year loop. Everything is changing. I'm looking to change work. Moving. Sense of misery, unhappiness. Lack of self-worth. Not doing anything worthwhile. I have to do something worthwhile. Isolated, cut off, lost. Directionless. 10-year cycle. Re-invent myself'.

H. 'Cut off'?

P. 'Busy with lots of people. Emotionally cut off. Numbness. Don't feel loved. Life's about connection only. Not unhappy alone'.

H. 'Connection'?

P. 'Emotional/intellectual. Understanding more than the words'.

H. 'Not connected'?

P. GESTURES. 'Distant. Flow . . . Not confident. Unloved, unvalued, not wanted personally or professionally. I'm on a mission, it's difficult without that'.

H. 'Unwanted by people'?

P. 'That's how I feel. Social life is busy; inside I don't trust it. Detached instead of plunging in. I'm observing myself, seeing myself like that. Inside I'm aware of it, rather than getting on with life. Detached and quite confused. I've a very strong feeling that the pattern of my life is disengaged. Living in a silent community. The ultimate path of human development is to end up as pure spirit. The challenge of sustainable development; no carbon footprint. Forsaking physicality. I understand that very clearly. A philosophical stance, that is the ultimate aim; as a path for living it is difficult, one is not an island. I'm not ready to jump off, to be a perfectly spiritual being'.

H. 'A spiritual being'?

P. 'A place of no physicality whatsoever. It's ultimately where the human species has to go. Physical and busy – that's not very clever. If we're intelligent, we'll ultimately go to the place of no physicality'.

H. 'Qualities of that place'?

P. 'I would not be. Pure light: my solution for most things! (She laughs). I'm obsessed with light. A place to live with lots of light, not a stone cottage. To see the sunrise and sunset, the sweep of life, and distance. A site to build a straw-bale house; it feels like the next step, but I've no idea how to accomplish it. Other people would have the same buoyant feelings'.

H. 'Buoyant'?

P. 'A bit busy. Great calmness and connection. Basic elements. You know where you are in your being. Completely connected'.

H. 'The opposite'?

P. GESTURES. 'A dark hole. Not feeling. Emotionally disconnected. Not calmly part of this world. The opposite: In the moment; in the landscape; I'm in exactly the right place and moment. Calm and strong. Bits of you are there, you need to get a lot more of it. It's similar to meditating. And a sense of being more in the community, socially'.

H. 'The feeling there'?

P. 'They are appreciating you, glad you are there; you are not just an extra person in the room, you have a place'.

H. 'Not appreciating'?

P. 'Isolation. Aware of myself; not sure I'm really here; distanced. Wondering inside why I am feeling distanced. I'm weeding cabbages. Disappointed in myself. Messing myself up. It taints the conversation. Sometimes a sense that I am acting out the part of someone who's weeding the cabbages, and chatting with Paul or whoever's on the farm. Un-relaxed. There's an underlying anxiousness; that's what the thyroid's about'.

H. 'What do you feel'?

P. 'Not at rest. Distant and too self-aware. Observing myself'.

H. 'Not at rest'?

P. GESTURES (Raises shoulders). 'Very aware of my posture. I've done 35 years of yoga. I'm not properly open in the upper chest or face; frown lines'.

H. 'Anxiety'?

P. 'I'm starting to go round in circles. It's because I'm not relaxed, I'm observing myself. Over-awareness leads to a lack of spontaneity. Need to avoid diminishing my own life in order to help others. Irony. I'm studying Embodied Knowledge with academics. They are struggling to pull themselves out of over-focused research, it's such a partial understanding. Need a full sense of understanding'.

H. 'Fulfils?

P. 'As a completely non-academic person, as a practitioner, they start to value my contribution. I'm really alive on those days. I spark. Affirming. Intuition. Planes of being'.

H. 'Spark'?

P. 'Together. Body and senses focused, alert and alive'.

H. 'Spark'?

P. 'Life. People are aware of me and I'm alive and present'.

P. 'A tiny bit about being in performance. Warm, alive. Connection being there together: you don't need to say a word. I'm sparked, I'm stimulated, interested as part of the group. A need for affirmation; a sense of place. What the hell am I supposed to be doing in this world? Time to move on, but I don't know how to evolve'.

H. 'How does it feel'?

P. 'Familiar'. GESTURES. 'Overlap while something new emerges and takes over. I don't have a sense of where I'm heading, it's not clear. I'm ancient: I will be 58. Sad and disconnected; I've got to accept all this. Standard view: this is the end: retirement. I'm not into that. There's no distinction between my life and my work. Coming up to 50 I was falling off the edge. I thought I was going to die. The challenge of the end of one of these clear cycles.

I'm capable of being cheerful, how people expect me to be. I'm better now at saying to people that things are not quite right. Ten years ago when I had cancer, I had big decisions to make. The second time I had radiotherapy. It came back again. I didn't feel as if I'd been defeated. It was a huge test of the way I was handling things; it stimulated changes and moves. A good dose of illness does you good: it's a challenge'.

H. 'Tell me the feeling'.

P. 'I'm very grateful for being. I was ignoring. Pushing. A big shove into not ignoring any longer. My thyroid may never be the same again'.

H. 'And now'?

P. 'I will see the endocrinologist in two weeks. They'll want to put me on something to calm this down. How will I ever know who I am if they want to poke me? Chicken and egg. Me; the thyroid causing me to feel glum?

At the cancer clinic I was having trouble with my left arm (breast cancer was on LHS). X-ray showed arthritis. Blood test showed overactive thyroid. They told me four weeks ago. It's clearly been kicked into action. I had virulent flu at the time. Since then my bodily functions have been disturbed. Thyroid got kicked at that point, may now be settling a bit. No wonder everything is racing (GESTURE: Waves hands very fast horizontally at chest level). I was hungry but couldn't eat. I've lost a huge amount of weight in one and a half years, and more recently with flu'.

H. 'Now'?

P. 'A slight sense of tremor. I've been struggling with my yoga. Tremor and problem with balance in yoga. The breast lump popped out when it needed to wave a flag (GESTURE). Big flag, Look here! A smaller flag on the outside, but a deeper, less superficial problem. It's about deeper things. Three days ago I started IOD 6'.

H. 'Your temperature'?

P. 'I used to be chilly, but in the last couple of years I've been wearing fewer clothes. Radiotherapy age 50 and menopause. I was bleeding a lot during menopause. I sailed into a slightly new place'.

Rx: Neon 200C, single dose

Quotations from the patient that guided me to Neon:
- 'Forsaking physicality.
- The challenge of the end of one of these clear cycles.
- The ultimate path of human development is to end up as pure spirit.
- Time to move on; I'm not clear how to evolve.
- Connection; being there and with you; you don't need to say a word.
- Not calmly part of this world.
- Great calmness and connection.
- The sweep of life.
- Pure spirit.

- Another ten-year loop, everything is changing.
- A sense of being more in the community socially.
- Overlap while something new emerges and takes over.
- Living in a silent community.
- It's like meditating.
- I'm in exactly the right place and moment.
- What the hell am I supposed to be doing in this world?
- To see the sunrise and sunset, and the sweep of life'.

Phone call June 8, 2007
I was prescribed Carbimazole 20 mg daily. They think if I take it for a short time, it might do the trick.

Follow-up July 9, 2007
P. 'How am I? (Pause) Better. But I know all the worries and bother have sunk further below the surface; I know they are there, but not with me quite so much. I'm pottering with this and that, cheery, finding something to do. It's easy then to think that everything has gone away, but it hasn't. Haven't answered the big questions. Who am I? Where am I going to? What am I? Who loves me? Who am I going to love?

I'm not quite so anxious; things to do meanwhile. I'm much more animated. Spirit is closer to the surface. Spirit and passion and stuff: that's nice. Engage; respond. Difference between alive and dead.

Something else: deciding what I want to work at. Polarities at the moment. I read my journal. Two paths: Yoga and moving into stillness. I could end up moving into a silent community. The other path: working as a community activist. Alert and alive. Campaigning. Trying to get a group together. Those two in some ways are in opposition. A sense of trying to hold these two things; one supports the other. GESTURE It's perplexing. Don't know what to do. Go much further west and just be. Or the other says "You'll die of loneliness". Be brave? Something new? Go to deepest Shropshire and watch the sky'.

H. 'If you didn't'?

P. 'Not having been brave enough to go and do it; sense of carrying on. Pending. Waiting for life to begin. Gemini's are terrible about decisions, we see things from all sides. I don't know what I'm deciding about'.

H. 'What are you feeling'?

P. 'It's with me all the time. A bit insecure. I'm not whole-heartedly into things. I think that's the right thing to do. Work is repetitive, there's a need to change. The dynamic of change is more with me. Getting on with ordinary things is dull. New York, emails. This year I want something exciting to happen and it hasn't yet. Or, coming to terms with the fact that there is no excitement. Irrevocably disappointed or mature and wiser and realising that stillness is not about exciting. Stillness and excitement. I can do some amazing things and have solitary spaces in between. The issue of a future direction. Lots of things to do is a smokescreen.

I started Carbimazole on June 8th. Had a blood test a week ago, no result yet. I ran out of it three days ago. I want to see what the blood test says, whether it shows it's almost back to normal. It's given me a huge appetite. I'm reluctant to take more Carbimazole, they suggested I take it for two months. My stool got firmer once I had been on Carbimazole for a week and I have less gas.

Rx: Wait

September 20, 2007 I receive a letter from my patient

Excerpts from her letter:
Hospital tests show her thyroid to be near normal: she is reducing the amount of Carbimazole. She writes: 'How I feel about myself has changed. It has been a wonderful gift to feel appreciated, maybe even love, after twenty years of being solitary. Surprised hardly begins to describe it! I think it makes a big difference. Time will tell. That was some remedy!'

Follow-up on December 18, 2007
She reports:
P. 'I reflect all the time. It's been an extraordinary few months. There is still a slight restlessness. I don't know where my home is. I've been very busy working – excellent, cheques coming in. What am I really doing now? Where am I going? I'm not half so bothered. I'm very happy with my man. We see each other only once a month. There's a sense of well-being. It's an enormous gift. I see myself in an appreciative way, it's bloody wonderful. I'm still able to look at my life and see how lucky I am. I'm lovable, maybe for the first time.

I'm much calmer. That equals more healthy, less undermining. I'm happy with the idea of just hanging about. A less driven Me. Growing old with a bit more grace. It's still going on, whatever you triggered'.

H. 'You and your thyroid'?

P. 'Pills are holding the thyroid in check. The overwhelming anxieties aren't pushing through. I still harbour an aspiration to be a super-human; a full soul; the urge to be one'.

Follow-up on May 26, 2009, after two and a half years

P. 'Last year I was bedevilled, knowing I had strong feelings for S. The issue was the physical manifestation of emotional turmoil. The universe delivered! Did I have the courage to be more receptive? I just knew. I had to completely let go. Everything's been different since.

The relationship: now it just **is**. I'm calm. I smile a lot now. More confident about just being me, the person I am'.

H. 'The silent community'?

P. 'It's a lot further back in my head. Things are not so polarised, I'm quietly getting on with things. The silent community is not for right now; when I'm 80 maybe'.

Comment (JS)

Other than the indications for Neon which Hazel has clearly listed, there are a few comments to add. Of course the relationship of element number 10 to the 'ten years cycles' is interesting, though, in itself, anecdotal rather than indicative.

The patient is isolated and emotionally cut off. There is no sense of connection to life, she is detached instead of plunging in. She feels it is time to move on, but she is stuck. All these could fit any of the nobles. However, there is a water-based metaphor – *'One is not an island'* (even though she lives in a silent community). Additional indications for Neon are the feeling of being very grateful for existing, and the desire to 'watch the sky'.

What is interesting is the yearning for the first period, Hydrogen and Helium. This is expressed as a desire for the ultimate path of human development, pure spirit, pure light; *'I am obsessed with light'*. Most indicative of this desire is: *I still harbour an aspiration to be a super-human; a full soul; the urge to be one.* Here we see the Neon half-soul yearning to join with its twin soul and return to the Helium undivided soul, pure spirit.

CASE 12.11 Attention deficit (hyperactivity) disorder

Matthias Strelow, Hamburg, Germany

Boy, age two

First consultation

The boy had been given the following diagnosis: perinatal asphyxia with damage to the brainstem, which showed two centres of hyper-conduction on the EEG. He had also been diagnosed with attention deficit/hyperactivity disorder with autistic tendencies.

The boy's muscular system was highly hypotonic and his coordination defective. He often stumbled, had to touch everything and wasn't able to cross-coordinate. Furthermore, he was unable to perceive positions, distances or the location of his body parts in three-dimensional space. So, for example, he couldn't crawl underneath tables or chairs without getting stuck, because he would perceive imagined obstacles.

His speech was inarticulate and he sometimes stuttered. It was difficult for him to comprehend what was said to him. A later examination showed that he could only process 20–80% of what he heard and suggested that he would always be severely dyslexic.

His mouth was always slightly open. He was unable to maintain eye contact and when looking at a person, always looked slightly to the right or above them. He had a peculiar high-pitched squeal.

He used bribery ('If you do this for me then I'll do that for you') to get as much as possible for himself. He complained a lot and demanded everything, but wasn't satisfied with things once he got them.

He didn't like to be touched. Whenever his mother tried to comfort him, he would push her away.

He annoyed his mother by urinating in different places. He interfered with many things because of his anxiety. However, he always treated his little sister solicitously in spite of their many rows.

He had a nervous cough at night that came on as soon as he lay down. He had chronic diarrhoea and undescended testes.

The symptoms became unbearable as soon as he ingested milk or chocolate. In contrast to his normal behaviour, he was quiet and shy in the presence of strangers. He was afraid of the dark (3) and needed light to fall asleep. He was also afraid of animals, especially of dogs (3) and insects (3), which made him panic.

Past history

When pregnant, his mother experienced uterine bleeding in the second month, which was treated with Sabina. She said: 'I thought the baby would leave and without the treatment he would have left.' At that time she was in a difficult relationship. Her husband spent the money on drinking and gambling, which made her panic. She developed fears concerning her existence and an indeterminate fear that something bad would happen. Her mental state alternated between euphoria and affliction. Throughout the pregnancy she experienced contractions and pressure towards the vagina, as if she wasn't able to hold the baby inside her. She finally delivered prematurely in the 34th week. It was a breech birth. The boy was immediately brought to the intensive care unit with severe neonatal jaundice.

From the beginning, he cried and moaned day and night other than when he was breastfed. He suffered from colds with clear discharge and had some kind of oedematous tissue. Throughout the first year of his life, his eyes suppurated and discharged gooey mucus. In the 4th week, he developed an inguinal hernia on his right side.

Cravings: eggs (3), sweets (3), dairy products (1), meat (2)

Analysis

Until January 1999, I tried several remedies without success including Vipera, Calcarea-carbonica, and Stramonium. I decided to re-interview his mother. She had previously told me about the boy screaming at night, but I hadn't understood the full extent of this behaviour. The boy would wake up and scream for about 2–5 hours and would barely respond when approached. His mother would have to stay in the room with him but wasn't allowed to touch him while his sister wasn't allowed in the room at all. I was baffled! How come I had missed such dramatic, persistent behaviour? I wondered whether my misperception was an analogy to the boy's perception disorder. The fact that he was unapproachable during these attacks confirmed his autistic tendencies and made me think of the inert gases, which don't combine with other elements. When asked about the boy's response to neon light, the mother said: 'It always makes him freak out. But only neon light has this effect on him, no other light'.

Rx: Neon 30C

Follow-up six months later

Since the first prescription, he hasn't had any nightly screaming attacks. His eye-hand and eye-foot coordination have improved. The hypotonia of his muscles has completely gone and he now closes his mouth properly. His speech is more articulate and he doesn't stutter anymore. He now knows where his different body parts are and has stopped touching everything. He listens to his mother when she tells him to do something and for the first time, made eye contact with her when she addressed him. He has stopped bribing people. He doesn't need light anymore to sleep. He has started to sing and make rhymes. He has stopped urinating in inappropriate places and no longer panics when taking showers. It is interesting to note that he used to dress up as a cowboy, in dark robes or in some other disguise. He no longer conceals his personality in this way.

The dry cough, which used to appear before his screaming attacks, got worse initially before disappearing entirely. In July, 1999, he had worms. When he failed to respond to Cina, I went back to Neon 30C and the worms disappeared.

Further prescriptions: During these months, two EEG check-ups showed clear improvement. However, the remedy only ever acted for a short time. I attributed this to the organic brain damage and therefore prescribed Neon LM3.

Follow-up four months after Neon LM3

The boy has started to wet his bed again at night. He has developed two big warts on the soles of his feet. He is afraid of owls eating him. When he was little he used to talk about owls being outside his window.

Rx: Neon LM3

Follow-up two months later

The warts have disappeared and so have the owls.

Analysis

The unusual family history seems to me to be the key to this case. The grandfather (on the mother's side) was sentenced to prison for homosexuality in the early years of his marriage. This was a big shock for his wife, who had no concept of homosexuality at all. She fell into a state of depression and never fulfilled her sexuality with her husband. However, she has remained married to him until this day despite his total refusal to take part in family life. The boy's parents were divorced in 1997. One year after the divorce, the mother discovered that she was attracted to women. The boy's mother subsequently told her ex-husband that she was attracted to women and he also admitted to homosexual tendencies.

Synopsis

To build a true relationship and allow an encounter between the 'I' and the 'you', one must first develop one's own identity. In my opinion, the fact that the boy dressed up and took on different identities suggests much about the central theme of Neon. However, it is still too early to draw definitive conclusions.

The boy played an important role in the dynamics of the family. His grandfather called him his 'prince' and started to participate in family life only after the boy's birth.

Comment (JS)

For me the most fascinating aspect of this case is the patient's existence in the second dimension of surface (See Case 4 and Chapter 10): *He was unable to perceive positions, distances, or the location of his body parts in three-dimensional space. So, for example, he couldn't crawl underneath tables or chairs without getting stuck.* The boy's inability to cross-coordinate is a further indication of lack of three-dimensional perception.

The autistic and backwards tendencies indicate that the boy is stuck in early developmental stages. His addiction to his own simple needs, resorting to bribery, show a two-dimensional personality controlled by desire and its satisfaction (like the drunk and gambling father). The constant sense of discontent is a strong indication for Neon, as is the mother's alternation between misery and euphoria during pregnancy. The boy was most likely treated with neon lights for the severe neonatal jaundice. These neon lights later caused the child to 'freak out'.

The excellent result in this case, including the improvement in coordination, dissatisfaction and the nightly screaming, provides useful clinical additions, as does the strange obsession with owls.

CASE 12.12 Fragility means to give an image of stability

Roberto Petrucci MD, Italy

Male, age 22

First consultation

The patient had several troubles: from the physical point of view, stomach and abdominal pains, slow digestion, diarrhoea and muscle cramps; from the psycho-physical point of view, frequent urination due to anxiety; diagnosis of border-line disease.

The patient came to visit at our centre when he was eighteen and he was visited by a colleague who prescribed based on the repertorial rubric 'BLADDER – URINATION – frequent – anxiety; from' which contains the single remedy, Hydrogenium, but the prescription of this remedy did not bring any benefit to the patient.

After six years, the patient decided to return to visit the centre; this time his psychiatrist sent him directly to me.

I asked the patient if he had ever consulted a homoeopath and he said no; I did not tell him that I had his old file; at the beginning I thought he wanted to hide something (this could also be a symptom). He started to tell me about his story and he said 'I feel a very strong body tension and I need to urinate very frequently and this is something that bothers me and it has a very strong impact on the quality of my life. I'm looking for something that creates a bond in me because I feel as if I'm divided into four parts: body, mind, language and emotions and this is essentially since forever; emotions are similar to atmospheric agents that come and go; it is like seeing the emotions flow, emotions are like water flowing under a bridge, I see them from above, but I am not involved in emotions. I always was anxious and when I was fifteen years old I started mixing alcohol and drugs'.

During the consultation he gave me a lot of information that I was able to divide into issues.

One important issue concerns the issue of time that he often mixed with the themes of memory and immobility; for this group of remedies the keywords are: denial of action, rest, sleep, quiet, inactivity, inert, detachment, forgetfulness. These were his statements about it: 'I live the emotion of the moment. The most recent emotion is the one I'm experiencing right now, I'm a little bit agitated; the fact is that I'm video-recorded and I'm going to listen to these words in the future . . .'

I asked him 'What do you give relevance to? What is your mission in life?' and he said: 'My mission is to be myself, to be peaceful, calm, unperturbed.'

He is an artist and musician; he said, 'For me music is a right, I like to fall into a trance, music allows me to cut myself off. This means to forget about myself, about everything, to have the memory of one who does not remember. I have to remember the instant I'm living; when I play music I lose my body. When I play music, I have everything in my mind, even if I play one note every fifteen minutes, and in fact this is what I would prefer'.

I asked him 'What is power for you?' and his answer was 'Power means not doing anything, power is the will of doing nothing. I feel tired, as if I was exercising aerobically all the time and also playing music is an intense effort'. (He plays contrabass and sometimes he plays one note every fifteen minutes!)

'I can be very detached from things. I forget about eating'.

I asked something more about alcohol and drugs. 'I started to drink alcohol and to use drugs when I was fifteen years old, perhaps because I'm a fragile person'. I asked him to explain fragility and he said 'Fragility is giving an image of stability, a fixed image but I always change . . .'

Normally, for 'fragility' we might take the rubric 'MIND – DELUSIONS – body – brittle, is' (Des-ac, Falco-p, Gard-j, Ign, Lac-leo, Nux-v, Sars, Seq-s, Stram, Tax, Thuj) But every symptom needs an explanation and here the patient said, 'I always change, I'm not stable, I don't want to give an image of stability, this is fragility for me'.

He showed me his artistic works: he closed books with some plastic and nails because he said that he is working on the theme of files, on the archive, on the container, on the memory.

I realised that all these words have a meaning for the group of the noble gases.

He also said 'I'm a person always with their head in the clouds, I frequently lose contact with the earth, with the soil. I'm more the sky, I have no roots, I feel borderless. The feeling I have about my body is that it is going to burst, to explode, but it's limited because we have to face the restrictions of our physical life. The air is wind, is freshness, air is also chaos, confusion . . . there is freedom; I believe that air contains the elements of life. The sensation that I have about my body is something burning, something frying, something sparkling, boiling. I have the sensation my body may dissolve'. Here we have a rubric from Synthesis: 'MIND – DELUSIONS – dissolving, she is' (AIDS, Ham, Neon, Olib-sac).

I think that in this case we have to consider the themes that come out from the words of the patient: *instantaneousness, instability, time, rest, borderless, sparkling, boiling, movement.*

Rx: Neon

Follow-up
The prescription of Neon gave a very strong amelioration of the physical troubles and an extraordinary change on the mental level. The patient said that he is no more divided, his work was more continued and he did forty-four concerts in two months!!

Also, the frequent urination disappeared and it's very interesting to realise that my colleague prescribed Hydrogenium, another gas.

Comment (JS)
As in Cases 2 and 6, we once again see the physical and watery aspects of Neon, urinary symptoms and diarrhoea, which disappear after the remedy. This reflects the emotional theme of Neon, which is expressed as: *'Emotions are like water flowing under a bridge'*. Most important is the *'sensation my body may dissolve'*.

Of particular interest is the strange sensation of being *'divided into four parts'*. The themes of division and even numbers are prominent in Neon (Case 9). Interestingly, the mention of 'four parts' and 'bonds' is reminiscent of the Adamas proving, Neon's counterpart in the second period (see Chapter 9, Angles of the periodic table)

The issue of time is also a prominent feature of this case and of Neon, especially the aspect of being in the Now: *'I live the emotion of the moment'. 'The most recent emotion is the one I'm experiencing right now'.*

The sense of detachment and the use of drugs and alcohol are repeated Neon features. Once again see the Neon separation from earth (Cases 6 and 7): *'I'm a person with their head in the clouds, I frequently lose contact with the earth, with the soil. I'm more the sky, I have no roots'.*

CASE 12.13 Premature birth

Camilla Sherr, Tanzania

This 9-year old girl was born at 24 weeks; her twin brother didn't make it and she almost died 11 times. She was translucent when born, all the organs visible through the skin, the size of a palm. When I met her she was living in her cocoon, not interacting, not knowing how to play, never hungry for food. She was extremely un-coordinated and had no 3-dimensional vision; hence she couldn't play or do anything involving balls.

After Neon she is playing rounders and tennis. She has friends. She is learning at school like any other kid. She now eats on her own and asks for food when she is hungry. She laughs and plays and is learning social behaviour. She is a different kid altogether.

CASE 12.14 Calm nature lover

Yossi Tagori, Israel

Woman, age 36

First consultation
Mother of three, Hydrotherapist.

Impression: Calm, Speaks quietly, thinks before answering, very pleasant and lucid. When she called for first consultation she did not ask the standard question people often ask before an appointment. She simply called and said 'I would like to come for a treatment'.

'For two years, since the last time I gave birth, I suffer from rashes and itch all over my body. I'm burning, really suffering, my hands are swelling. It comes every day, I took all kinds of medications but nothing helps me.

People think I'm shy or maybe even snobbish, but the truth is I have no need to connect, I feel fine with myself.

Cannot bear lies and politics, I can be promoted at work but then there will be a need to manage and deal with people, and I do not have that desire .

I would love to leave it all behind and go to a long trip to the countryside. I love walking in nature, touching the earth, feeling the body struggle, the physicality of it. I can see the all diversity of colours in nature.

Since childhood I always turn off the light when showering, I cannot stand a strong light, prefer dim light .There will never be a fluorescent light in my house, they drive me crazy .

Food: Aversion to the white of the egg, aversion capsicum.

Love hot and dry weather, desert wind.'

No repertorisation was made. Her calm and self-contented nature made me think of a noble gas. Her aversion to florescent lights made Neon seem to be the appropriate remedy (Neon is the only noble gas repertorised under 'Light agg') Florescent lights are sometimes named Neon lights (although florescent lights mostly contain argon and krypton, but my prescription was based mostly on the patient's nature) . The main issues were her contented character and the desire to ground in earth and nature. There were no Helium issues of whether to enter into this world or not, no body and soul issues. There were no Argon issues of amusement and the enthusiastic-laziness axis.

Prescription: Neon 30c

Follow-up six weeks later
'The day after the remedy I experienced a great relief, rash and itch drastically reduced and I felt something open up. Then there were days when rash and Itch came and went, but much better overall. It is clear to me that my body came back to life and there is a healing process. Recently I started to remember dream.'

Prescription: Neon 200c

Follow-up six weeks later
'The rash is almost completely gone, I feel a profound change in me. I suddenly look at myself, it creates conflict between me and my

husband. I have to put my needs ahead. I finally enrolled in gymnastics team.'

Follow-up six weeks later
'Rash and Itch completely disappeared. I feel like my life is going through profound change, Thoughts and desires I buried inside are coming back to me, I have returned to life.'

Between meetings I came to understand that patient was not taking the remedy upon my instructions. She told to me that: 'I know the right time for me to take the remedy and the right time to stop'. I agreed for her to continue in this way.

Comment (JS)
Note her occupations as a hydrotherapist on one hand, yet seeking to connect to the earth on the other. Also important are the NBWS giving birth, the itching and ailments since giving birth. The typical noble gas aversion to lies and desire to be alone are also present. Though she has a content and enlightened view on life and seems very connected to her truth, there is also something of a two-dimensional personality. After the remedy she discovers the third dimension, sides that have been buried in her.

CASE 12.15 Second prescription

Jeremy Sherr, Tanzania

Female, age unknown

First consultation
The following case is that of a lady who had many remedies over many years, with good success. Overall, she has done very well and has been cured of very serious pathology. I present this as one of the follow-up consultations she has had along her homoeopathic journey, as it has some interesting information to offer.

Her last remedy was Jade, several months ago.

'Feeling as if I am two years old and younger. My mother would leave me and say she was never coming back. My heart felt on hold and broken, I didn't know what to hope for or what to feel. It is hard for me to love someone who might never be there again. I never knew if to grieve or hope.

I fell in love with someone married who disappeared. Deep grief. I can't sleep or think due to the grief.

If I go near the ocean I get vertigo, I can't tell where the sky ends and where the earth begins. Everything moving – tides, moon. The moon aggravates, I can't feel where the earth is, I can't handle gravity. I sit and look at the moon in the water, a magnified moon.

Subliminal feeling of cancer in the vagina or urethra, like I can smell it.

Radiation sickness after a local tsunami. Feeling of dematerialising. Radiation from cell phone aggravates, I feel it in my bone marrow. Very electrical; if I touch things I see/imagine blue light. Light explodes into blue light. Everything is much worse since the tsunami. Very sensitive to earthquakes. (she lives in a volatile region of the world.) Not sure what is me and what is the planet and what is humanity.

Lost like a little child. Splitting myself between two things.

The main things at the moment: water, radiation, grief.'

Rx Neon 30c, one dose

Follow-up five months later
'Doing great! I am the happiest and healthiest I have been in my life.

Two days after the remedy all of a sudden I felt the earth! Before, the earth was puzzling me with her gravity. Now I feel like being in the womb of the mother again, the universal mother.

After that nothing happened but everything happened! All the grief I had about my mother vanished, I was bonding with the Great Mother. For the first time in my life I bonded with the Great Mother, it was really easy. Like finding another part of myself. Then many gentle and beautiful things happened! My relationship to numbers changed, before I always preferred 3, now all the numbers are my favorite. I started to like more colours than before – before they were jarring to me, all the red and orange and blue and green. Now, I am easy with them. Many other beautiful things happened, I got a lot of recognition. All of a sudden I could manifest things that could never happen before.

My relationship with time changed. Since I was small I made mistakes in time; I could not tell the difference between past, present and future; I did not understand what was past or present. All the time issues in me corrected, I could just be; I just was, flowing in a beautiful way.

Things changed in my health. I could run for the first time in my life; before, my knees would swell and bleed. I started to run; now I can run two hours without trying or breathing hard, I became a spiritual runner.

All of a sudden I found many close relatives and felt miraculously protected by the universe. Feels like all my generations and ancestors are being healed. Like a great protection. Many things became possible, Everything I was always wishing for my whole life.

I think I'm growing up, moving my attachment from my mother to the universal mother.'

Rx: Neon 30c, when needed

Patient continued to do excellently for long time, all was great.

Comment (JS)
I am particularly fond of second prescriptions, which reflect the true nature of clinical practice. This woman, after many years of a healing journey through homoeopathy and shamanism, finally arrives at the crucial moment of being two years old, the point at which her mother deserted her. Here she is stuck, lost like a little child in a state of unresolved grief; a grief which repeats itself throughout her later life.

In this state, the watery essence of Neon rises up, a tsunami of emotions. Her aggravation from the moon, the ocean and the tides, her lack of ability to separate earth and sky, are all strong indications for this remedy, as is her sensation of being split between two things. Her sensitivity to electrical energy, and images of blue light, add colour to the picture.

As we have seen in previous cases, the solution to the watery Neon predicament involves finding the earth, feeling the gravity of the universal mother, and with this, a change in perception of time, numbers and colours.

A beautiful clinical confirmation of the Neon proving.

CASE 12.16 'It is only me here and now, light and nothing else'

Roma Buchimensky, Israel

Female, 26 years old

First consultation

Diagnosis: different psychiatric disorders including schizophrenia.

Her mother brought her to consultation.

She communicates-answers questions but it feels like she is not completely awake and aware of what is going on around her, more concentrated on her inner worlds.

She has two major problems-weakness, lack of concentration.

She repatriated to Israel from Ukraine alone and in the beginning was ok, functioned normally and independently. For some time she tried to make it herself, but her condition slowly got worse and she became a social psychiatric case.

'I cannot function normally. I didn't get out of bed for years. I was lying in bed. I have schizophrenia. I have stones in my bladder. I was recommended a surgery. Voices and visions pursue me.

I behave weird. My behavior doesn't suit the surrounding. Those multiple visions and events are with me.'

(*I asked her to describe her character*) 'I am an introvert, I wanted to be a psychologist. I wanted to learn what kinds of people exist and how it is possible to help them. Person's soul is a mystery. It is interesting to uncover secrets. People, characters, reasons for such or such behavior when they are conscious or unconscious. Psychological help in choosing a partner is also interesting. When their characters don't suit, it is a reason for fights and divorce. In order to live in peace, people need to suit each other. It is important that people have a family so that they are not alone.

Happiness is being confident in myself, it is when you are satisfied and you communicate, love, friendship and good financial situation.'

(*I asked her what is the opposite, when you don't have all this?*) 'Lonely, frustrated, sadness, lack of desire to live, to drown, to hang yourself. Easy death.'

(*What do you like to do at your free time?*) 'Read books. I like bad literature.'

(Tell me more about yourself.) 'I am not patient, positive, confident of myself, even snobbish, introvert, good-hearted and I was full of joy.'

(Fears?) 'Darkness, Monsters'

(Tell me how you were as a girl.) 'Full of joy, helped at home, communicative, confident, but at the age of 13 I started to get distant from people, straight forward.'

Prefers cold, like juices – apple, grape, pears, apricots. Likes salads, meat

Aversion: fish

Likes sweet and sour and to sleep on stomach *(was said spontaneously).*

Repeating dream: in high school she dreamt that she climbs up the tree and falls down. It happened at the same place every time.

She takes psychiatric pills.

(I asked her to say the most important complaint) 'Lack of concentration. It is not pleasant to be not smart enough. Lack of concentration doesn't let me live in this world.'

(I asked her again about fears.) 'Fears: big insects, spiders, snakes.'

(I asked her about hobbies.) 'To read fantasy stories.'

(I asked her to be more specific about her bladder problems.) 'Sharp and strong pains once in two weeks.'

Her mother tells: that she lives inside herself more than outside. From early childhood: weakness in hands and need to lie down all the time. Like she closed herself up and if there is a problem, she tries to solve it alone.

Observation: when her mother talks about her, she calls her 'little girl' (she is 29 years old now).

Rx: Neon 200c, one dose

About the remedy choice:
Someone very naive. Constantly needs help. Doesn't make it alone in this world. Introvert, inside of herself, feeling not suited to the world.

She is in a situation of pre-family, pre-relationships, but is lonely. On one hand, she wants communication very much, on the other hand she keeps distant from people.

She said about herself-simple and straight forward.

What her mother added, suits the remedy: weakness in palms is weakness in ability to do. Palms symbolise the ability to do something in this world. She still cannot be alone/independent in this world. What is characteristic for the row of noble gases is the will to solve the problem alone (she is not able but tries it anyway).

Follow-up one month later

'After the remedy I felt fresh, felt better.' One week after the improvement she fell down to abnormal world. But she felt her abnormality less and the visions were not sharp. She dreams more often, more physical weakness.

Rx: Wait and watch

Follow-up one month later

Rx: Neon 200c, one dose

Follow-up one and half month later

After she took a remedy, she felt instant improvement in her condition, both mentally and physically.

Mother added: 'My little girl has much more energy now. She started to watch movies, she went back to reading. She started to help at home. She can watch a movie for 40 minutes without a break!'

Follow-ups every two months

Repeated doses of Neon 200c.

Follow-up March 2011

Increase dose to Neon 1M

Follow-up November, 2011

Increase dose to Neon 10M

Follow-up May, 2012

Neon LM7 with subsequent increases to LM 9, 11 to current dose Neon LM23.

Follow-up October, 2014

During all these years she came to the clinic with her mother, and the last time she came to follow-up alone (distance more than 100 km).

She has a part-time job: she helps handicapped people to participate in projects.

Since she is treated with homoeopathy, she didn't have to take any allopathic pills for her bladder pain attacks and also diminished slowly the doses of psychiatric treatment.

During last year-year and a half there were almost no complains about the bladder.

A 'journey' meditation

During one session in April 2014 I did a 'journey' meditation with her. (She repeated 'we'– mom and me. Her mom also repeated 'my little girl'.)

(*I asked her to describe, What is us?*) She closed her eyes and said: 'Us is mom and me.'

(What do you like?) 'I like juice.'

(What is juice for you?)

'Juice is freshness, pleasant coldness, sourness and sweetness. Freshness is a feeling that embraces you and brings positive feelings. It is nice and joyful. It is something new. I have a feeling that very good change is going to happen really soon. That something interesting will come. It is a feeling of youth, health, power, filled with energy, the whole future is filled with light and joy.'

(Tell me about the light.) 'Light is what gives light and all that gives light to our lives. Everything that brings satisfaction and joy.'

(What is joy?) 'Joy is when you get what you dreamt of.'

(What is new?) 'New is a change for better. Everything changes and becomes new. Freshness and joy.'

(What is light?)

'Enlightened. Light takes with it all the evil and brings enlightenment and joy. This light is good. It is clean. It is gentle, caressing, it gets inside everything. The light circulates in a body, it is yellowish with a bit of greenish.

Stillness, rest, freshness, softness. It is only me here and now, light and nothing else.'

She started the 'journey' meditation with 'Us' and finished by 'It is only me here and now, light and nothing else'.

Synthesis of cases

The themes in the cases above represent a nice collection of symptoms which taken together represent the clinical picture of Neon. We find an abundance of watery images and idioms, with an affinity to the moon, sky, ocean, ships, ice, tsunami and the urinary system. These watery images often include a lack of clear connection to the earth. The Neon patient floats in a world with no boundaries, a world in which sky melts into water, mother dissolves into child. In this world the thin layer of a two-dimensional firmament provides the only solid division between these homogenous entities, and he clings to the two-ness it creates; for the spiritual world of 'one' has been left behind, an unattainable light fading into the distance. Neon must come to grips with a divided world. And whilst the even division of this water-world provides some comfort, it lacks the solid ground on which he may stand with his own two feet. He longs for his mother's overflowing uterine waters to break, so that he may burst free and stand on the earth. It is from this earth that the child, like a tree, may grow, developing a three-dimensional personality, the 'I' of an adult identity.

Enter Day Three

Clinical observations

Louis Klein, Canada

JS – I am grateful to Louis Klein for contributing the following observations from his study of the proving and from clinical practice.

Very adept at mathematics.
Incredible memory for dates, numbers.
Effects of jobs that require mathematical calculations.
Mathematical idiot savant.
Focus on even numbers and the number two.
Gambling – Las Vegas.
Idiot savant.
Making lists.
Highly scheduled, even small events.
Routines.
Loss of contact.
Alzheimer's disease.
Live in the moment – 'free'.

Childish.

Loss of ability to cope.

Passive.

Retreating.

Spacey, nothing can make an impression.

Beyond right and wrong.

Confusion around daily events in the moment.

Motionless feeling.

Cut off from relationships (and emotions).

Has a hysterical and excitable partner who compensates for lack of contact and emotional expression.

Absent-minded.

Helplessness.

Effects of institutionalisation or incarceration.

Impractical.

Inability to nurture or provide emotional support.

Dwells on past disagreeable experiences.

Unafraid of death.

Loves to drive a car.

Colours.

Dreams of vivid colours, rainbows.

Love of sunsets.

Photography of sunsets, colours.

Bright clothes, environment.

Dreams of birds, flying.

Delusion someone is knocking at the door.

Expect police to come to the door.

Feeling they are about to be attacked.

Poor recognition of people.

Down's syndrome, Asperger's syndrome, Autism.

Naïve.

Worse modern living.

Anachronism, old fashioned.

Anorexia.

Faintness on rising.

Reaction to overuse of psychedelic drugs and marijuana.

Can appear intoxicated.

Worse neon lights.

Ailments from neon lighting.

Neonatal jaundice.
Desires natural environment.
Worse noises of radio and TV.
Ailments of newborns.
Joint pain.
Injuries last long.
Lower back pain and sciatica.
Ailments from sitting long.
Carpal Tunnel Syndrome.
Sensitive to heat and cold or completely insensitive.
Pain in temples.
Sensation of constriction in head.
Better hot bathing.
Ailments from head injuries, motor vehicle accidents.
Warts on fingers.
Awkwardness.
Anorexia.
'Breatharians', desires no food, or minimal food.
Sensitive to the smell of cooked foods.
Overeating.
Craves fat of meat, salt.
Exhausted on descending stairs.

13

RELATED AND SIMILAR REMEDIES

Nobles

All the nobles can take a direct vertical route to each other, rather than the roundabout route through the horizontal periods. Their similar natures will become apparent as we progress through this series.

When the noble gases align, there is an express connection between them, and we can progress directly from one to the other. This is revealed in the provings, but I have also observed the relationship between these remedies in clinical practice where the noble gases often follow each other well.

From a philosophical point of view, one might say that the seven nobles were created first as complete elements connected by a direct line, and only later did all the other elements appear to fill the gaps between them. Helium, in particular, has a close affinity with Neon.

Helium

The following are Helium symptoms that relate to, or are shared by, Neon.[1] Knocking on door, didn't go to open it.

Keys broken in locks.

Delusion at night that I could hear the phone ringing or a knocking on the doors.

Second or fifth day, take us back through timeless state (the angels do all the praising and adoring on the second day and on the fifth day they do all the work). The second day ones were like archangels.

Sensation of slipping over on ice.

Out in the snow, excited by emerald heads of mallards, I felt like a duck on ice.

In my inner vision I could see stars that looked like snow, and snow that looked like stars, falling very gently. Ameliorated by silence and the purity of snow.

Complete the web. Enter the mirror, dive into watery reflection.

Morning – dawn the opening of a radiant eye. Felt Neon was seeing the eye but Helium was seeing through the eye.

Yet before the waters of emotion, Queen of the heavens, honouring her King.

Leaving the waters of home? We grow towards the light.

I was in some Japanese-inspired surroundings. An egg-shaped pond with ice cold water, and a thin layer of ice on top. I didn't know if it was muddy or full of plants, fishes, other creatures, or anything dangerous. I undressed completely and jumped in after a short hesitation. The others around thought it was a great, impressive, respectful thing to do. My body broke the ice as I jumped into the pool. The water was ice cold but clear. I went all the way to the bottom, and then rose slowly upwards. The sun was shining through the water making all the bubbles glitter. I had to take a deep breath while still under water, and found that I could breathe in the water. When I broke through the top it was like going through a membrane. I rose from the pond feeling like a new person, a cleansed person, actually more 'me' than ever. I was in contact with all of myself, and felt very whole. It felt like an initiation, and I was met with deep respect afterwards. Right next to the Japanese garden was a farm with a square swimming pool like an American pool. People were swimming, screaming, shouting, laughing and acting rather hysterically, thinking they were having a great time. Some of them had been drinking. It all seemed very superficial compared to the quietness and spirituality right next door. But I felt I was a part of them too – or they a part of me. I knew what I wanted, and how I preferred to be, and which part of me I wanted to live. When undressing to go into the pond I felt very shy and naked; on rising from the pond the nakedness was spiritual in a way, with no shyness.

Naturally, Helium shares many aspects with Neon, parts of which overlap. At times they can be difficult to differentiate clinically from each other. This relationship can be seen in Case 12.10, and will be further elaborated in the following chapters.

Oncorhynchus tshawytscha

Salmon often swims in Neon waters. I have found that these two remedies are related and follow each other well. Here is a narrative from the proving of Oncorhynchus that illustrates the connection.[2]

I am alien on land. At this thought my chest feels compressed and my breathing is difficult and anxious. Like resistance to breathing at birth, air feels dry with burning lumps. On the sweet perfume of foetal water, no wonder I would not be bound. Power, knowledge stripped at birth. Skill of fluid movement lost. Sounds so sweet, I was all ear. Sound pervaded my world, tenderly massaging my body. Infinite knowledge and bliss, a place of fear unknown. No need to come up for air, weightlessness, blueness, no day or night, a time to play in the watery space. A transition from the heavenly realms. Sirius, ancient memories stir, tears as salt as the oceans flow, I return to the ocean. The ocean of bliss. The sun appearing the same size as the moon. The moon with the power to draw the tides, soon to feel your fullness.

Jade: Alignment of the Tai Chi master

There are several other remedies that portray the concept of vertical alignment with 'the Force'. One of these is Jade, the most noble of precious stones, known to unite heaven and earth.[3] To my mind, Jade relates to the noble gases and to Neon and Argon in particular. Jade is mentioned several times in the Argon proving. The following Jade symptoms clearly illustrate some points of similarity with Neon.

Economy of motion. No extra movements. Like a cat.

My muscles feel strong and toned, flexible and powerful. I'm invincible. From inner strength.

I have a direct line into the truth.

If you keep everything in alignment nothing will ever drop!

I feel very powerful and very strong. If I am in this position (upright-JS), no one can hurt me. I feel very centred, it would be very difficult for anyone to get me off my centre.

This is why the Chinese do Tai chi. It is the perfect movement all the time, moving around your own axis. I feel invincible!

A feeling of superiority which comes from the knowledge that this is so much better. If someone is out of alignment, they are so much weaker. This is a mega inner strength.

This is like a feeling that I know exactly who I am, what I want, why I am the way I am. Complete sense of power from being aligned, from being in the place I am supposed to be.

If anyone practiced being in this position they would be invincible. It forces you to be in a straight line and is a place of power and strength.

This is the positive side of Jade. At worst, Jade, like Neon, suffers from desire, dependency and addiction. It is interesting to note that the vertical alignment of Tai Chi, mentioned in the Jade proving, is achieved by bending at the knees and thus straightening the spine; servitude that leads to mastery and freedom.

Polaris

Another remedy that relates to the vertical line of stillness is Polaris, or the North Star. Directly above us, Polaris is in line with the heaven-earth axis,

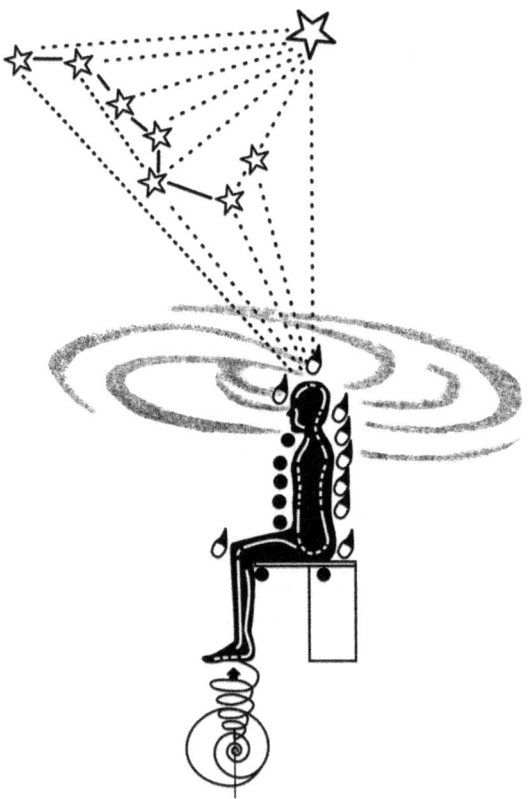

Figure 13.1 Diagram depicting Chinese North Star alignment meditation

pointing the way to the sky window. As I mentioned previously, stars feature strongly in Neon. Here are some examples from the proving.[3]

A sensation of internal stillness, with energy bubbling, alternating with the desire to laugh at the slightest movement.

I felt this stillness and when I kept perfectly still, I felt so in balance and at peace and alive. It was enhanced when I physically didn't move a muscle, it got better.

When you move out of the centre there is a very fast movement.

A real sense of timelessness, very still and very happy to be here yet not wanting to move or create a change in that.

Iridium

There are several similarities between Iridium and Neon. These include a relationship to numbers and colours, a noble and graceful nature and an association with the iris.[4]

Iridium is the peak element of the 6th period. If the periodic table is depicted as a spiral, iridium is positioned opposite the nobles, reflecting something of their nature. The following is a list of related symptoms from the *Synthesis Repertory*:[5]

MIND – CHILDISH behaviour
MIND – DELUSIONS – alone, being – world; alone in the
MIND – DELUSIONS – angels, seeing
MIND – DELUSIONS – awakened; he is – just been awakened; he has
MIND – DELUSIONS – beautiful – landscape; of
MIND – DELUSIONS – body – lighter than air; body is
MIND – DELUSIONS – born into the world; he was newly
MIND – DELUSIONS – born into the world; he was newly – wonder at the novelty of his surroundings; and was overwhelmed with
MIND – DELUSIONS – clouds – black cloud enveloped her; a heavy
MIND – DELUSIONS – clouds – reach the clouds; he seems to
MIND – DELUSIONS – diminished – all is
MIND – DELUSIONS – dogs – he is a dog
MIND – DELUSIONS – emptiness; of
MIND – DELUSIONS – enlarged – tall; he is very
MIND – DELUSIONS – floating
MIND – DELUSIONS – floating – air, in
MIND – DELUSIONS – messenger; she is a
MIND – DELUSIONS – mystic hallucinations

MIND – DELUSIONS – narrow; everything seems too

MIND – DELUSIONS – new; everything is

MIND – DELUSIONS – objects; about – bright objects; delusions from

MIND – DELUSIONS – objects; about – shining

MIND – DELUSIONS – rainbows; of

MIND – DELUSIONS – separated – floating in his inner self; he is

MIND – DELUSIONS – strangers – surrounded by

MIND – DELUSIONS – water – under water; he is

Aqua marina

Given its watery nature, Neon naturally resonates with some of the other water remedies. For example, the following Aqua marina symptoms remind us of Neon.[6]

Impression of being spied upon.

Fears that others are watching him working; during bath feels that bathroom door is open.

This is related to fear of being penetrated personally. They will close the curtains to avoid being seen. [Mangialavori]

Feels himself tormented, distracted, agitated.

Tormented by lascivious thoughts, with the fear of becoming mad; tries to find his peace in religion.

Anxiety.

Ameliorated by fast motion; riding in carriage; perspiration; ice cold drinks; cool open air.

Hypersensitive personality. Unable to pass urine in presence of others.

Strong aggravation from company.

Sense of religion, especially to reduce strong sex drive. [Mangialavori]

Aqua marina has been principally used for the effects of living near the sea [such as biliousness, constipation, headache, etc.]. [Clarke]

Fluoric acid

I have already mentioned the similarity between Neon and its periodic neighbour fluorine, which, in the form of Fluoric acid, has excessive energy and muscular ability, and is able to exercise without any fatigue (think marathon runners, triathlon wallas and compulsive gym rats).

It would be also be interesting to compare lithium fluoride with neon, as it seeks to emulate neon in the number of electrons. Not much is known about this element other than that LiF crystals are more transparent to short wavelength ultraviolet radiation than any other material. It is used in optics, for windows, prisms and lenses; in nuclear reactors and radiation detectors.

Jan Scholten describes this remedy as 'naively entering the world of glamour'.[7] Farokh Master has added it to the rubrics 'egotism' and 'inconstancy'.[8]

References

1   Sherr J. *Dynamic Materia Medica: Helium*. Glasgow: Saltire Books, 2013.
2   Sherr J. *Dynamic Provings Volume 2*. Malvern: Dynamis Books, 2002.
3   Proving by Sherr J. See www.provings.com and www.dynamis.edu
4   Sherr J. *Dynamis Provings Volume I*. Malvern: Dynamis Books, 1995.
5   Schroyens F. *Synthesis 9.2 Repertory* RADAR 10 Archibel Homeopathic Software.
6   Vermeulen F. *Synoptic Materia Medica 2*. Encyclopedia Homeopathica Archibel Homeopathic Software.
7   Scholten J. *Homoeopathy and the Elements*. Encyclopedia Homeopathica Archibel Homeopathic Software.
8   *Synthesis Repertory*. RADAR 10 Archibel Homeopathic Software.

14

NEON: ANALOGY, BIOLOGY, COSMOLOGY

The following chapters expand into analogy, geometry, philosophy and poetry. The understanding of these concepts may allow greater comprehension of Neon and the periodic table and their application to more subtle and difficult cases, as well as offering a peek at different perspectives. The practice of homoeopathy involves the practical application of analogy and metaphor to the art of cure. One never knows where the clue will come from, and it is good to train our minds to be perceptive and flexible in this regard. If this is not your game you may safely stop here, as the knowledge of symptoms, essences and cases gained from the previous chapters will suffice in practice. If however, you enjoy travelling to new dimensions, I invite you to join me on an esoteric voyage beginning in Flatland, bursting through the ozone layer and proceeding to nearby planets, distant galaxies, the seas, the Bible, movies, poems, genetics and an orchard.

Flatland

In 1884 Edwin Abbott, an English schoolmaster, wrote *Flatland: A Romance of Many Dimensions*,[1] in which he used the analogy of a two-dimensional world to criticise the class discrimination that was prevalent in the Victorian era. The book retains its popularity today because of its exploration of dimensions. The following is a synopsis. For a more in-depth understanding of dimensions I recommend reading the whole book.

The characters live in the two-dimensional Flatland, and so they are all geometrical shapes. Flatland society is very hierarchical: the narrator, a teacher, is a simple 'Square'. Noblemen appear as circles, men are polygons, soldiers are triangles and women are mere lines (which also renders them invisible from certain angles and highly dangerous).

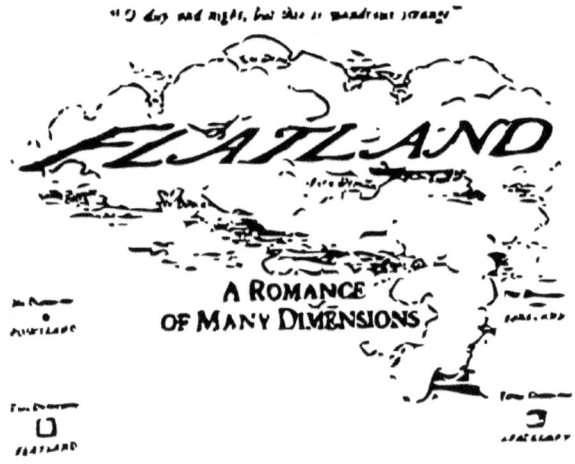

Figure 14.1 *Illustration from* Flatland

The book opens with a description of Flatland:

> Imagine a vast sheet of paper on which straight Lines, Triangles, Squares, Pentagons, Hexagons, and other figures, instead of remaining fixed in their places, move freely about, on or in the surface, but without the power of rising above or sinking below it, very much like shadows – only hard and with luminous edges – and you will then have a pretty correct notion of my country and countrymen. Alas, a few years ago, I should have said 'my universe': but now my mind has been opened to higher views of things.

The Square, a mathematician and a very lawful citizen, goes out of his way to explain to his grandchildren that there is no such thing as a third dimension. But when he is visited by a Sphere from 'Spaceland', he finds it hard to deny that a heretical third dimension exists. In a dream, he pays a visit to the old 'Lineland', but the king and queen of that country refuse to acknowledge his existence because they cannot imagine that there could be any dimension beyond a line. Finally he visits the Sphere in Spaceland, where he is able to experience the third dimension personally – something he never thought possible when he lived in Flatland.

After the Square's mind is opened to new dimensions, he tries to convince the Sphere of the possibility of a fourth (and fifth, and sixth . . .) dimension. The Sphere is offended and sends his student back to Flatland in disgrace. The Square then has a dream in which the Sphere visits him again, this time to introduce him to Pointland, the land of the first dimension, the line. Pointland is ruled by the King who is a Point, who is unable to accept that there is a land of two dimensions and believes that the Square is a voice in his own mind. The Square then tries his best to convince the rest of the two-dimensional Flatland shapes that there is a third dimension, even though they can't see or imagine it. No one believes him, and his heretical efforts land him in jail where he spends the rest of his life trying to convince others that the third dimension exists. The poor Square is the only entity in Flatland who knows the source of light:

> I alone in Flatland – know now only too well the true solution of this mysterious problem; but my knowledge cannot be made intelligible to a single one of my countrymen; and I am mocked at – I, the sole possessor of the truths of Space and of the theory of the introduction of Light from the world of three Dimensions – as if I were the maddest of the mad!

I find this book to be a fine analogy to some of the states we have examined in our exploration of the nobles, from the one pointed pre-hydrogen singularity, to the linear Helium and the two-dimensional, surface-bound Neon. Consider the following passage, while bearing in mind the sceptics of homoeopathy.

> Then put yourself in a similar position. Suppose a person of the Fourth Dimension, condescending to visit you, were to say, 'Whenever you open your eyes, you see ... a Fourth Dimension, which is not colour nor brightness nor anything of the kind, but a true Dimension, although I cannot point out to you its direction, nor can you possibly measure it.' What would you say to such a visitor? Would not you have him locked up? Well, that is my fate: and it is as natural for us Flatlanders to lock up a Square for preaching the Third Dimension, as it is for you Spacelanders to lock up a Cube for preaching the Fourth. Alas, how strong a family likeness runs through blind and persecuting humanity in all Dimensions! Points, Lines, Squares, Cubes, Extra-Cubes – we are all liable to the same errors, all alike the Slaves of our respective Dimensional prejudices.

I suggest that in future we substitute the word 'sceptics' with 'Flatlanders'.

The Flammarion engraving

The wood engraving shown in Figure 14.2 is known as *The Flammarion*. This illustration is considered to be a representation of medieval cosmology, a metaphor for the scientific and mystical search for knowledge. The artist who created the original engraving is unknown. It was first published in 1888 in Flammarion's book *L'atmosphère: Météorologie Populaire*.[2] with the following caption:

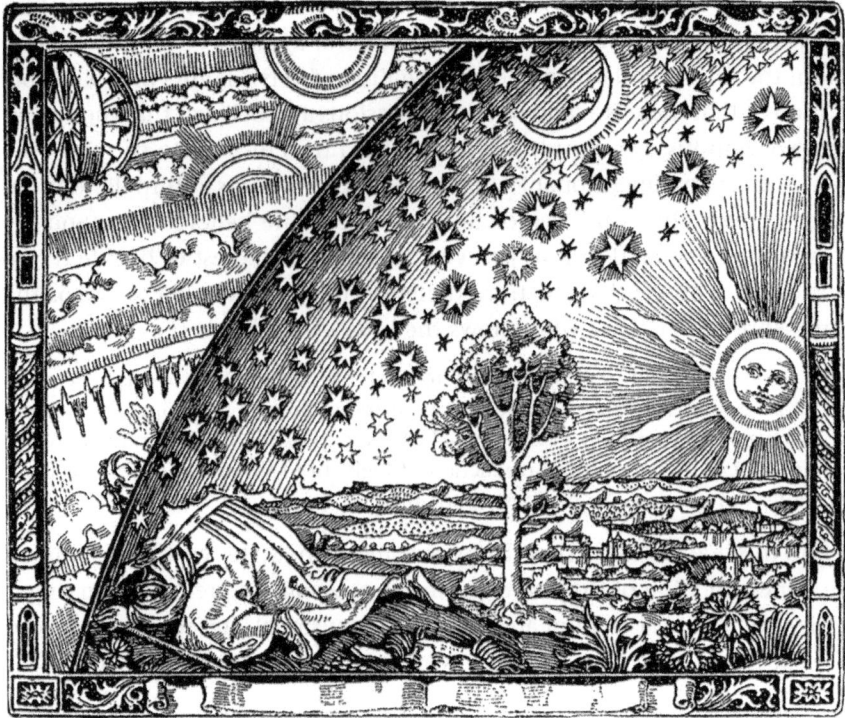

Figure 14.2 The Flammarion engraving[2]

'A missionary of the Middle Ages tells that he had found the point where the sky and the Earth touch'.

The Flammarion portrays a flat earth with a starry sky or firmament above and a man poking his head and right arm through an opening in the sky. Having penetrated the firmament the man can see multiple layers of 'clouds, fires and suns beyond the heavens' and a 'wheel in the middle of a wheel' as described by the prophet Ezekiel in the Bible. This reflects our understanding of Ozone as the firmament that separates the material world from the heavens, a cosmic egg that humanity has succeeded in penetrating.

Stars, planets and quasars

There are some curious symptoms in the Neon proving that demand further examination. Themes include certain deities, planets, quasars, elements and their relevant mythology. We begin with a look at elements from the following symptom:

Walking up a long gradual incline, I felt I was covering great distances with every stride. I felt I was doing the usual 20-minute walk in seconds. I felt like a Titan in seven-league boots, but then I couldn't decide which league boots they were and I wanted an even number. My thoughts went titan-titanium-uranium-Uranus-clouds-clouds-where is the sky?

This strange proving expression makes us question the link between Neon and the concepts of Titan-titanium.

Titans, titan and titanium

The word 'Titan' and its derivatives represent great size, strength and power, sometimes resulting from a direct connection between heaven and earth that we can associate with Neon.

'Titan' represents something gigantic and powerful, as in the 'Titanic'. In Greek mythology, the Titans were a race of extremely powerful deities who ruled during the Golden Age. They were born from a direct connection between sky and earth: Gaia (Mother Earth) fell in love with Uranus (Father Sky) and gave birth to the twelve Titans. It is interesting to see that the deities Helios and Oceanus (Sun and Sea) are among the Titans.

Some scholars believe the word 'Titan' to be related to the Greek verb τέμνω (to stretch). A Greek poet wrote, 'But their father Ouranos, who himself begot them, bitterly gave to those others, his sons, the name of Titans, the Stretchers, for they stretched out their power outrageously'.[3]

Titan is also the largest moon of Saturn. It bears a strong resemblance to Earth, with smooth lakes and rivers of liquid on its surface, along with ice and rocks. Its thick, humid atmosphere is similar to what scientists believe existed in the Earth's early days.[4]

Finally, element number 22, titanium, lives up to its namesake. Titanium is as strong as steel but weighs much less. It is also very resistant to corrosion.[5]

Uranus and uranium

How do the proving expressions regarding Uranus and uranium relate to Neon? Uranus, a huge, icy planet, is the seventh planet from the sun and the third largest in our solar system. Unlike the other planets, it tilts to the side, so that it rotates on a horizontal axis. The planet was named after the Greek god of the heavens and sky. In mythology Uranus was both the son of Gaia, the Earth, and then, her husband. He became the father of the

Titans and the grandfather of Zeus. After Uranus' castration by Cronus, his son, the sky (Uranus) and the earth (Gaia) separated.[6] Astrologically therefore, Uranus represents the breaking down of rules, patterns and structures. Out of this destruction comes change, creativity and new inventions.[7] We can relate this to the newness of Neon.

Uranium, a silvery-white metallic element, atomic number 92, was discovered in 1789 and named after the planet. A radioactive element, it is used to create electricity and to fuel nuclear reactors. Within the earth, the continuous decay of uranium produces so much heat that it is one of the causes of convection and continental drift.[8]

Just like the relationship between Titans and titanium, Uranus and uranium represent the Neon dichotomy of sky and earth, contrasting heavenly bodies and powerful gods with the equally powerful earthly elements and mortals.

Seven-league boots

Originating from French fairy tales, 'seven-league boots' impart a magic ability to walk seven leagues (21 miles/34 kilometres) with each step. In one stride the wearer is able to cover the distance a normal man could walk in a day. In the stories, the hero receives the boots to help him achieve a goal or perform a superhuman feat. The phrase, characterising exceptional speed and ability, once referred to horseback messengers. Galloping between coach houses, they only touched their boots to the ground every seven leagues when changing horses.[9]

Summary

The proving expression *titan-titanium-uranium-Uranus-clouds-clouds-where is the sky?* depicts the relationship of heavenly bodies with their earthly namesakes, the gods of heaven and earth, Uranus and Gaia, the planet Uranus and the element uranium, the moon Titan and the element titanium. If the clouds are the barrier, where is the sky? If we can only penetrate the sky-barrier and unite the heavens with earth we will receive god-like power, becoming Titans with seven-league boots.

Tilts

The following 'symptom' opens new avenues that deepen our understanding of Neon, the first being the tilt of Uranus.

Doing research on Uranus, I found that the planet has a tilt. For 42 years one side is in the dark and then it comes into the light for 42 years. Uranus feels very near, like a friend. The quasars are much further out and it was a real stretch for me to go so far.

The fixed tilt of the axis of a planet is what determines the cycle of seasons. Seven of the planets in our solar system spin like a top, with axes that are oriented almost perpendicular to the Sun's orbital plane. The Earth has a 23.5 degree tilt. Uranus, however, is tilted at an angle of 98 degrees, which means it spins on its side around a horizontal axis, with the polar axis facing the sun. This causes the poles of the planet to have 42 years of continuous sun and 42 years of continuous darkness. Only a thin band at the equator has a short cycle of light and dark. During the equinox when the equator faces the sun, its light/dark cycle is similar to the Earth's.[10]

One possible interpretation of the symptom analogy is that Uranus, with its intense tilt and long cycles, signifies the split of light and dark. Hence Uranus, named after the god of the sky, relates to the first day of creation in the Bible and the first period of the periodic table. Neon yearns to reconnect to the first period, but it lies at a tilt and cannot penetrate the window of the sky, other than when it is in vertical equinox.

Quasars reflect the Neon theme of difficult connection with the heavens as the proving symptom 'quasars . . . a real stretch too far'. Quasars (quasi-stellar radio sources) are faraway, massive, compact, spiralling objects that surround a black hole. They suck in gases, stars and galaxies and absorb their energy, to create a burst of radiation and light thousands of times stronger than the Milky Way. As the brightest and most powerful objects in the universe, they are the most distant and therefore the earliest in the evolution of the universe.[11]

Dreamt of quasars again. From a distance they looked blue. There was a luminosity about them. Up close they were the most intensely bright things I ever saw, unbelievably condensed light, making the sun look like an orange in comparison. I knew nothing of quasars before this dream.

The genetics of incarnation

In the book *Helium* I examine the analogy between incarnation and meiosis, a special type of cell division that forms the sperm and eggs cells required for reproduction.[12] The final stage of this process relates to Neon and incarnation. To briefly summarise, the end result of the meiosis process is four gametes, sperm and egg cells, each ready to combine into a new

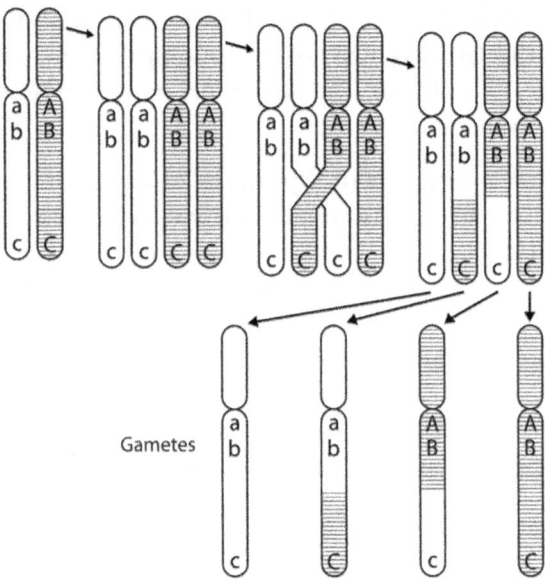

Crossing-over and recombination during meiosis

Figure 14.3 A schematic diagram of Meiosis

zygote composed of one paternal gamete (sperm) and one maternal gamete (ovum). These reproductive cells are haploid – meaning they contain half the amount of chromosomes of a normal body cell. Figure 14.3 shows a simplified description of meiosis.

The following is a simplified description of meiosis. (Figure 14.3)

DNA replication – each cell contains four strands of chromosomes. Each chromosome makes a complete copy of itself. (Four **individual** strands of chromosomes replicate, then pair up to make four **pairs** of chromosomes).

The pairs 'cross-over', swapping parts of their genetic information.

Two daughter cells formed – the four pairs of chromosomes divide, allowing each of the two pairs of the newly-mixed chromosomes to move into a daughter cell.

Four daughter cells formed – the pairs of chromosomes in the daughter cells separate, sending half of each (one chromosome) into a new daughter cell. Each new daughter cell now has half the normal number of chromosomes (haploid) and is a gamete – sperm or ovum – ready for reproduction. Thus when a sperm combines with the ovum at fertilization, a normal number of chromosomes for a human cell is created (diploid cell).

In the correlation between meiosis and the stages of incarnation, Helium relates to the first part of meiosis (Figure 14.4). Initially there are four original components of the complete Helium soul (four hydrogen nuclei or

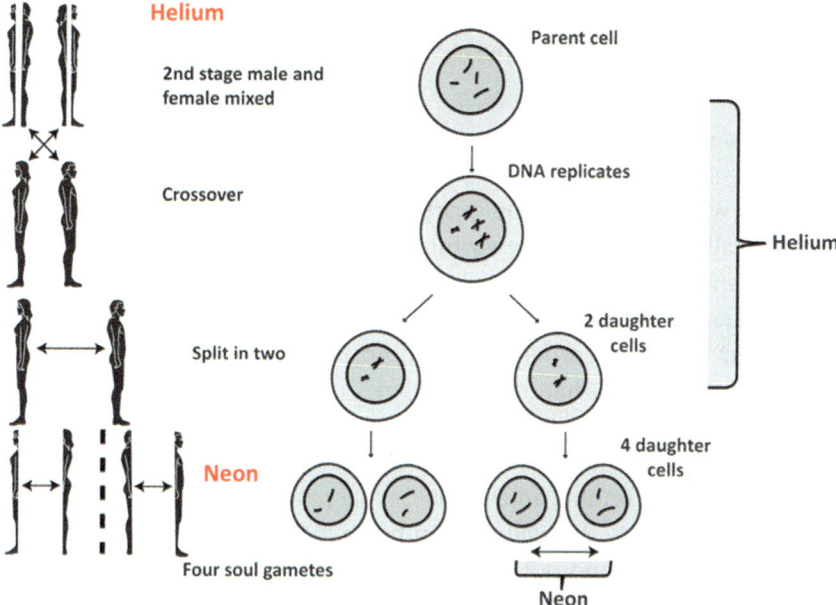

Figure 14.4 Meiosis stages corresponding to evolution of the soul in Helium and Neon

chromosomes). These combine in four basic pairs, which I name Male-yin, Male-yang, Female-yin and Female-yang. The four pairs recombine and cross-over in a variety of permutations. The process ends after the original four-part Helium soul splits into two daughter cells, representing two soul mates, each ready to incarnate in two separate bodies (corresponding to the two daughter cells in meiosis).

The final part of meiosis is analogous to the Neon stage of incarnation. The two daughter cells split into two haploid gametes, each containing half as many chromosomes as the original cell. This results in 4 haploid gametes. After the half-soul enters the body it splits into two halves (a quarter of the original soul). One half migrates forward to the eyes, the other half retreats to the shadows, and a firmament divides the two.

The end result of meiotic process is a single haploid cell, sperm or ovum, waiting expectantly for its other half, its soul 'ga-mate'. At first the gametes are tranquil but as the time of meeting grows nearer they begin to itch with desire. Certainly the ovum is reminiscent of the cosmic egg waiting to be breached. As we have seen in the proving of Neon, there are several references to ova.

I felt like I was an unfertilised egg, an ovum, very peaceful.

Felt like one of thousands of ova sitting there, waiting, with the thought that they were all female. They felt like they were there, complete and unfertilised.

When a woman is born, all her ova are ready and present. Their numbers are relatively few and the stock will not be replenished. Each ovum must patiently wait her turn in the ovary tower, until one day, in the distant future a gallant knight, riding a white horse with a swishing tail, will penetrate her membrane.

One question remains. If ova are so strongly represented in Neon, where are sperm? The answer will be found in *Argon* (the next book in this series).

Neon's 'light' front-half seeks its 'dark', posterior shadow side. If these two unite internally, an acute explosion of bliss and truth results, a healing fusion process. In chronic disease, however, we lean into life and seek to become whole by finding an external sexual partner, one that will emulate our other half. This is usually a non-healing fission process, because the solution is external and not internal.[i]

As we learned from the Helium proving, even if each half finds its true partner, the combination still represents only one half of a soul mate; two quarter-souls making up one half-soul; these are merely soul mates as opposed to twin souls. Our twin soul, the other full half of our soul, is hidden behind the firmament of our delusion and desire, and so may be difficult to find, even if standing right in front of us. We will only find it if we unite our two sides internally, becoming 'half-whole'. From there we can stand upright and penetrate our two-dimensional image of love.

And so, it is a long process back to the source. Nobody said it was easy.

DNA

In my book *Helium*[12] I compare aspects of the remedy to the process of DNA replication. (Figure 14.5) The double helix duplicates itself during the early stages of mitosis (cell reproduction), which results in two strands becoming four.

Neon corresponds to the first stages of protein synthesis in the cell, known as transcription. Through this process DNA sends the genetic message that instructs the cell to create proteins. Once a **new** cell is formed, it must synthesise protein. The **double** helix DNA **splits** into two strands, one leading strand and one lagging strand. These strands are **mirror images**

---

[i] For further explanations on this theme see *Dynamic Materia Medica: Helium*[12] and my teachings on acute and chronic disease.

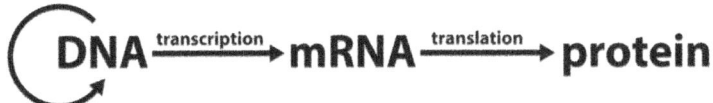

Figure 14.5 DNA replication, transcription and translation

of each other. Each strand is then copied into a **mirror image** messenger RNA. This mRNA migrates out of the nucleus and into the cytoplasm through pores in the nuclear membrane, where it will be translated into proteins, the building blocks of life.

Translation is reflected in the third and fourth periods in which the incarnated soul creates a material body around it. This process will be elaborated in the next two books of this series, *Argon* and *Krypton*.

The Bible, evolution of the soul and the second period Upper Water, Lower Water and Firmament

The proving of Helium led to my exploration of the Bible and Cabbala and to an understanding of how Helium relates to the first day of creation. I have continued this biblical analogy in my investigation of Neon, which, as I have demonstrated, relates to the second day of creation. On this day God places a firmament between the heavenly waters above and the earthly waters below. One of the issues that puzzled me was the relationship of the neon atom and the H_2O molecule to the heavenly and earthly waters. What is the correspondence between them and which element or molecule is analogous to the firmament? I wrestled with this problem for some time.

There were several possibilities, of which I list four:

1. The perfect Neon represents heavenly water and the cruder H_2O represents earthly water.
2. H_2O is both the waters above and below.
3. Neon is the firmament itself.
4. The firmament is something else.

For some time I believed that the first possibility was correct. Neon has the same number of protons and electrons as water, hence Neon can be viewed as an analogy of water. It seems logical to imagine that the perfectly symmetrical, noble neon symbolises heavenly water and that H_2O, the water of life, symbolises 'lower waters'. This theory is reinforced by the accounts of Neon provers, who experienced a blissful and direct connection with the heavens.

Furthermore, during cosmic evolution, while oxygen appears before neon, water forms after neon is created.[i] Hence, heaven before earth, Neon before water.

Water, however, was already created and present in the first day of creation. Before the second day the waters were one homogenous body, which must be H_2O. Perhaps neon represented the firmament itself, the dividing noble barrier between upper and lower waters? I was puzzled, and I remained puzzled until I realised that the firmament was Ozone.[ii]

The anomaly of the second day

Based on the proving of Neon, and the concept that each noble gas corresponds to one of the days of creation, I had assumed that Neon represented the completion of the second day.

However, the second day of creation has an anomaly. It is the only day of creation on which it is not pronounced '**and God saw that it was good**'. (Perhaps that is why no one likes Mondays). On all other days this sentence marks the completion of a day and its 'project'.

One common interpretation suggests that the 'water project' was not completed until the middle of the third day, at which time God separated water from earth.[13] On this day God pronounced 'It was good' twice, the first time after the waters are withdrawn to expose the earth and the second time after vegetation appears. In other words, only when the waters had been divided top from bottom and separated from the earth, finding their natural level, did God deem it 'good'. Hence, we could say that the 'water project' actually finishes in the middle of the third day. I will refer to the two parts of the water project as Water Project A (the separation of water above from below-Day Two) and Water Project B (the separation of water from earth-Day Three). Here is how it looks in the Bible:

Day Two – Water Project A

And God said: 'Let there be a firmament in the midst of the waters, and let it divide the waters from the waters'. And God made the firmament, and divided the waters which were under the firmament from the waters which were above the firmament; and it was so. And God called the firmament sky. And there was evening and there was morning, a second day.

Day Three first half – Water Project B

And God said: 'Let the waters under the heaven be gathered together unto one place, and let the dry land appear'. And it was so. And God called the dry land

---

[i] For full correspondence with Professor Carlo U. Segre of Illinois Institute of Technology on this topic, see Appendix.

[ii] See Appendix.

Earth, and the gathering together of the waters He called Seas; and **God saw that it was good.**

Day Three second half – Vegetation Project
And God said: 'Let the earth put forth grass, herb yielding seed, and fruit-tree bearing fruit after its kind, wherein is the seed thereof, upon the earth'. And it was so. And the earth brought forth grass, herb yielding seed after its kind and tree bearing fruit, wherein is the seed thereof, after its kind; and **God saw that it was good.**

If God's declaration '**It was good**' relates to the noble gas state of completion then Neon corresponds to the end point of water project B, the middle of the third day. In summary, **the second period, lithium to neon** (Figure 14.6), **corresponds both to** *Day Two and the first half of Day Three* **of** creation, the entire biblical 'water project'.

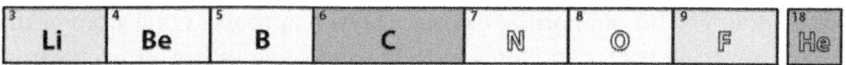

Figure 14.6 The second period

Which element then represents the complete firmament? From our earlier reasoning we learn that as this period progresses, the second dimension of surface unfolds until, by the end of Day Two, (Water Project A) the firmament is completed. This should occur somewhere within the second period, but before neon, which is already in the middle of the third day, at the end of water project B.

The firmament that God creates between heavenly and earthly waters can only appear after water is created. Water can only be created after oxygen appears; therefore the separation of water below from water above by the firmament can only occur *after* the creation of oxygen. Between oxygen and neon, we only have ozone (O_3) or fluoride to choose from. From a study of the proving of Ozone, it becomes apparent that we can equate ozone with God's firmament. I will begin, therefore, with an investigation of Ozone, followed by an exploration of Oxygen and Fluorine.

Ozone

(Note: when I refer purely to the chemical element there is no initial capital letter (ozone, oxygen) whereas the remedy name or esoteric concept of an element begins with a capital (Ozone, Oxygen). The boundaries here are often blurred and you can choose to understand these concepts in any way that suits.)

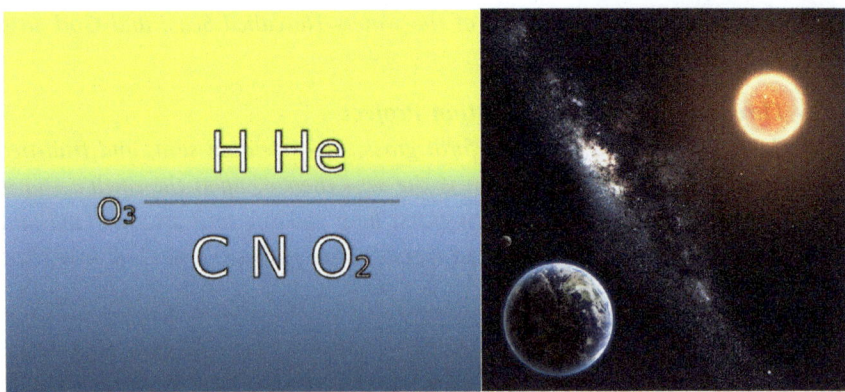

Figure 14.7 Ozone separates the intense light of the first period from the second one

The dark, pungent and toxic Ozone is essentially opposite to the colourless, odourless, life-supporting oxygen. Oxygen appears as one atom of the water molecule H_2O, two atoms in the O_2 molecule in the air we breathe, and three atoms in the ozone molecule, O_3. The atmospheric ratio of O_2 and O_3 fluctuates in response to solar radiation, temperature changes and other catalytic influences. Ozone forms a thin layer 20–50 kilometres above the earth's surface, which protects life from ultraviolet light and harmful solar radiation.[14] This ozone layer appears as the dark, blue-black sky we see just after dusk.

We might say, therefore, that in direct contrast to its sister oxygen, the dark ozone layer separates the first period of hydrogen, helium and direct sunlight from the second period of organic life (carbon, oxygen and nitrogen) and protects it from intense radiation (Figure 14.7).

. . . and darkness was over the face of the deep

Naturally, the Ozone proving is full of references to the colour black, and some to the opposing red or white colours. The following proving references are from Anna Schadde's Ozone proving and my own unpublished proving.[15]

Talks a lot about colours (red and black).
I imagine that the countryside is covered by a black, soft, warm layer of snow.
Dream a black spider crawls through the left corner of the mouth into the mouth.

The ozone layer is analogous to melanin in the skin. Melanin, derived from the word black, refers to insoluble pigments that account for the dark

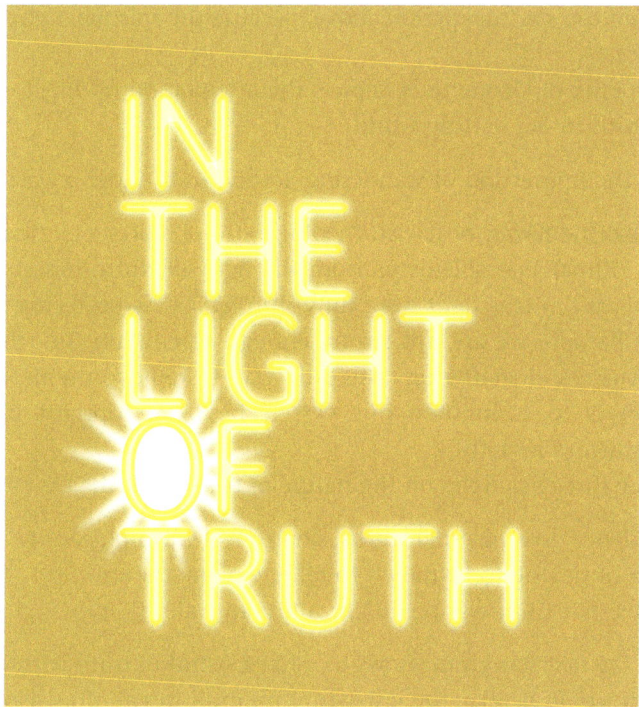

Figure 14.8 *UV Truth*

colour of skin, hair, fur, scales, feathers, etc. Just as the bluish-black layer of atmosphere shields the world from the direct rays of sun, black melanin pigments protect our body from excessive sunshine and radiation. We know that holes in the ozone layer lead to melanomas, a defensive attempt of the body to protect against increased solar radiation.

I have the impression of wandering around as if under a glass dome.

In most languages light and truth are synonymous. The phrases 'I saw the light', 'the truth dawned on me' and 'in light of the facts', are good examples of this relationship. Truth is a powerful force for good, as long as we are strong enough to accept it. Otherwise, truth can be extremely dangerous to mortals, hence we mostly avoid it. The truth is that we can handle truth but not *the whole truth*. If we do not filter universal truth, it kills us. If we were to learn all the secrets of heaven and earth we would fry like moth on a flame. We need protection from knowledge of the whole truth until such time as we are able to cope with it. Ozone is the filter, the firmament, the black lie that shelters us from a light and truth that is too powerful for us to handle. It is the screen that shields the organic second period from the spiritual period above, because the spiritual light of God is too intense.

The proving of Ozone thus depicts the attenuation of direct ultraviolet light or truth in our earthly world.

> I have the impression of wandering around as if under a glass dome.

In cabbalistic terms, or Jewish theology, ozone represents the dark shell or screen (Klipa) that shields us from the light of truth, but at the same time prevents our true light from fully shining. These protective shells are necessary because we are not strong enough to contain the whole truth without our vessel shattering. The only way to remove the need for this protection is to strengthen our vessels by being upright physically, emotionally and morally.

Here are three examples on the nature of truth from the Ozone proving:

> I experience great, eternal truths, depth; feel truth physically.
> Feeling of having to be direct, to tell everyone the truth.
> It seems that truth was being like a line in water (JS proving).

While the first symptom shows us what a world of truth without Ozone protection would be like, the last symptom indicates another aspect of the firmament or Ozone, the geometry of truth. At the equator, where the earth is closer to the sun and the angle of the sun's rays is perpendicular to the ozone layer, UV light penetrates the ozone layer much more directly. When we get closer to the poles, the light hits the ozone layer at an angle, and consequently penetration is much less intense. Hence, the need for a melanin-intense, black skin near the equator and pale skin in the north and south of our planet.

In a similar way to light, truth burns when told directly, but is attenuated when given at an appropriate angle. Ozone is full of references to the damage caused by too direct a truth, as opposed to the art of softening it. Here are some examples:

> Argument with mother. He told her the truth, not what she wanted to hear. . . . It burst forth out of him, the total confrontation.
> I feel secure, am able to lead more firmly. Gave a pupil a detention; something I had meant to do for a long time and saw as necessary but had never managed to achieve. Am surprised at how smoothly it went and was accepted. Good mood, feel strengthened.
> She finds it easier to refrain from criticizing. She wasn't bothered about her father eating noisily and her mother-in-law sniffling. Didn't even notice it. A feeling of 'They are already old, you can't change them.'

Girlfriend says that he is softer, not as stern and determined, not as impatient as usual. Normally puts forward his point view more harshly, now more calmly.

Opposing the theme of being direct is the theme of progressing at more gentle angles, which is also apparent in the proving.

Dream the road is tarmacked. I had to drive in swerving lines to make a path between the tarmac-machine and roller in order to get to the house.

Dream I went to the barber and he cut my hair horribly. It was angled cut, not a straight line. In my dream, my hair was jet black and extremely straight. (JS proving)

Here is another example of a 'black lie':

Guilty conscience on slaughtering a ram. 'I have a pitch-black conscience that I'm having the animal slaughtered.'

Initially this guilt seems a semi-noble emotion. However, we soon see that the 'black ozone guilt' is a compensation filter that protects us from the painful light of truth, which is that despite anything we may say or feel, we did kill the ram. Having a guilty conscience reduces this truth and makes it seem somehow justifiable.

The inner nature of Ozone may be wild, but it is tempered by a black layer that covers up and hides its wild characteristics.

Dream of dirty water, sea with wild big waves, but it is black almost like liquid tar. Someone says: you should see how wild the ocean is without tar. A 60 year old woman is sitting with her legs wide open so that it is visible that she is naked under her skirt. She is totally uninhibited.

Finally, Ozone has many dreams of climbing and descending mountains. The common theme that characterises these dreams is that it is hard to get to the top but easy to go down. In a similar vein, one could say that it is harder to live near the narrow peaks of truth then to fall into the polluted, but comfortable, valley of lies.

On a mountain with no proper path. The whole slope consists of sand, we can't continue.

Climbed a really steep mountain with two small children. I had to protect them so that they wouldn't fall down. It became steeper and more dangerous. There was only the possibility of ridge-walking on top. I got into a panic as to how to descend again until I had the idea to simply slide down. We got down safely.

On a journey. I'm standing on the plateau of a mountain and am frightened that I will fall over the low railings and fall off the mountain.

Dream went with a friend on a skiing holiday up to the top of beautiful, sunny, snow-covered mountains. On the way down he injured himself. It was a glorious place, this mountain top. It was so sunny and bright. Happy. (JS proving)

Dream I was at the top of a mountain. We were relaxing and having food lying around in the sun and chatting. My group was due to walk back down the mountain to their cars. . . . They left without me having forgotten that I was there with them. By the time I was ready to go it was late and it would mean I'd have to walk in the dark. (JS proving)

The ozone layer can move up and down dynamically. In today's modern world pungent, polluting ozone with its dark, black energy has proliferated on earth, while the upper layers that should be protecting us have developed huge holes, disturbing the balance of truth and lies. We are being exposed to knowledge we are not yet ready for while breathing the polluted air of daily lies.

The contrast between oxygen and ozone now becomes apparent. While oxygen connects the first and second periods, heaven and earth, by means of the water bond, ozone is the firmament that separates heaven and earth with a black protective screen of lies. In the stratosphere, Ozone protects us from the truth, but when its dark and smelly energy descends onto earth the result is a toxic mix of pollution and lies.

I am standing in the bath and having a shower. The shower attachment (metal) falls into the bathtub: a large black patch in the enamel. I apologise for the sloppy and dirty house with a black rim around the bathtub.

Ultimately, ozone is a necessary barrier to truth and light. When in the right place and quantity it protects us. When there is too much of it, too close to earth, we fall prey to its lie.

Feel connected to the dark forces (who are normally the baddies), with the culprits (of victims, persecution . . .). At the same time there is an incredible feeling of superiority towards everyone striving for purity, light, love.

This is the ultimate lesson of Ozone: It is our duty and wisdom in life to learn when and where to tell the straight truth and when and how to soften its angle. Telling a person too direct a truth can burn and kill, while a total lie will suppress. There is a more gentle middle path that we must learn to navigate. We learn how to receive truth and when and how to reveal it. With each truth we gain we grow stronger, climbing closer to the top of the mountain, where the paths are narrow and dangerous, but the view magnificent.

Oxygen

Oxygen, element number 8, is the breath of life. Oxygen forms a bridge between the first and second periods: by grasping two hydrogen ions it forms water. Symbolically Oxygen anchors the ethereal Hydrogen-based soul into the living body. Carbon provides the structure.

The following example serves as a metaphor for the role that Oxygen plays in our life and materia medica. We begin the journey with Hydrogen and Helium. As a reminder, please refer to the analogy of the whole Helium soul being a fusion of four Hydrogen soul fragments (or soul-gametes).[i]

The four parts of the soul combine and recombine in different configurations as they incarnate. This process begins with a heavenly combination of twin souls. The four parts then continue to recombine until they arrange themselves in a more earthly configuration of soul mates. Just before the soul enters the body it splits into two halves, two soul mates, each composed of two Hydrogen ions or soul fragments, our yin and yang aspects. Each half-soul enters a different body, or one remains outside of a body. These two halves yearn for each other throughout life. Because we enter this life as half a soul, the missing half must be temporarily replaced.

Oxygen, by forming a chemical bond with the half soul's two hydrogen ions, replaces the 'missing' half of our soul. Following a newborn baby's first breath (or intake of oxygen through the placenta), the Oxygen atoms bind with the half-soul's two Hydrogen ions, forming H_2O – the water of life. Water is therefore analogical to one oxygen mother lovingly capturing two hydrogen soul fragments into her watery womb.

In effect, we are now water; our body is composed of approximately 65% water.

At death, after our sigh, oxygen intake ceases, and the two captive Hydrogen soul fragments are released from the watery river of their Oxygen-bonded lives to float skywards and merge into Hydrogen clouds and the sea of souls.

By binding with the two hydrogen ions of our 'half-soul', Oxygen acts as a substitute for the other half of our soul, our missing soul mate. Oxygen becomes our 'life-mate'. While we can exist without water and food,

---

[i] To understand these concepts further, please refer to Sherr J. *Dynamic Materia Medica: Helium.*[12]

Oxygen is essential to our every breath. Our physical yearning for air is as powerful as our spiritual yearning for our soul mate; Oxygen, our mother and lover, serves as a temporary replacement for our essential 'other half'.

From an existential point of view, what does Oxygen's role as soul mate substitution represent? What feature do we not care about as souls, but desperately cling to in life, even until our dying breath?

In one word, Oxygen, the big O, is our eg-O.

Ego is the factor that our incarnated Oxygen-based soul possesses and that our Helium soul lacks. I refer to the proving of Oxygen by Dr Chetna of Mumbai to demonstrate this.[16] The following is a collection of ego-related statements from various provers, arranged A.I.O.P. (As If One Person)

I was an egocentric person. I had a lot of pomp about myself. It was as if I know everything. Only satisfying my ego, I wanted to be a person of great importance. I have a dream of making a big name where I will definitely make a difference to everybody, make a difference in everybody's life. It was all an ego-based creation. I used to think that I am the greatest person on this earth. I think that I am becoming my old egoistic self. My elder brother said that I am being egoistic. My ego was hurt. If you do not consider me, than that is the ego. I can decide for myself because I am independent. We are grown-up why should somebody else decide for us. They want people to satisfy their egos. Let people call me selfish, it doesn't matter. I have now realised that each person is important and unique in his own way.

And the icing on the cake:

'I have been born by a special birth, I am vayu-putri (the daughter of air, vayu=air).'

Oxygen midwife's us into the world of I, me and mine. There are three interrelated things that our ego craves most, love, recognition and money, and Oxygen represents them all. Let us begin with love.

Oxygen serves as a substitute for soul love, from mother to lover, and provides us with a romantic, blissful high. But high will often turn to sigh, for oxygen, derived from the Greek 'acid' or the Germanic 'Sauerstoff', can easily sour.

Love is like oxygen
You get too much, you get too high
Not enough and you're gonna die
Love gets you high
'Love Is Like Oxygen'[17]

Romantic love, represented by Oxygen, is a palliative surrogate to our soul mate, and our soul mate is but a proxy for the wholeness of our twin soul.[i] From the proving of Oxygen:

I was having thoughts of the purpose of our existence. What is the purpose of existence of us humans? This Deepak Chopra propagating love, how can you teach someone to love?

It is about my marriage. I feel I have chosen the right person. I wouldn't find a free **atmosphere** in an arranged marriage . . . a sacred arrangement. (emphasis mine JS)

Whatever love and affection was there, for me it is not there now. You don't consider me at all, it's like 'Just shut up, you do not have a right to talk'. 'You are no more of any importance to me'.

Sighing and crying deeply, sighing fast and deep, gasping for air, deep sobbing.[18]

Hence, we seal our love with a kiss, a mouth to mouth transfer of oxygen and body fluid.

The second ego-based factor that is prominent in Oxygen is the need for recognition and acknowledgment, to be seen as having value by others and a positive evaluation by others. Here are the provers' expressions:

They cannot take me for granted. I have some value in life. I am important and what I do or say has to be recognised, due value has to be given to me. You don't value me and you treat me like dirt. You can't take me for granted. I did not want to be where I am not acknowledged. It is as if you are here but you are not acknowledged, not considered. I am trying to make an effect on people, I feel that there is no appreciation. Everybody gives seminars, and gets appreciation. They should acknowledge my feelings also. My efforts should be acknowledged. I should be considered something. There was no consideration, no regards for me. I was not regarded at all. They are not giving me my due, my position, no respect. When you do work they don't value it, then why work for them. They are big because of the work done by us and they don't value it. Don't let your mom-in-law take you for granted. They are illiterate so they don't value education. I don't want to meet their expectations. If you don't value my opinion than you better continue the other treatment. I was thinking of about giving respect to each other and considering each other's sentiments and individuality. I have become very evaluative of people's behavior – this is more on the critical side. Nobody is so important.

---

[i] To understand this concept further please refer to Sherr J. *Dynamic Materia Medica: Helium.*[12]

Finally, the issue of value manifests as a strong regard for money:

I have been quite thoughtful while spending money. I travel by the bus and save money, and petrol and the environment in the bargain. I was a spendthrift. I have begun to save every possible rupee I can.

My mom lost a large sum of money – I told her this is a lesson for you to learn, now you will never misplace any money. You will learn to value the money.

We are consumers and we are very important. Only because we pay they are running the whole show. Through our taxes they get their salary paid.

Dream: As we come out, to the left is a beach, while to the right is a lot of poverty, there are slums. The scene is that of extreme poverty. On the beach you see a lot of fishes dying. They are being thrown on the shore and you can see them *gasping for air and water*. The whole scene is very horrible and depressing and the feeling is that as if the end of existence is coming. Towards the right there is a lot of poverty. People look very worn out without flesh on their body, only bones are seen. And the tragedy is that that behind the slums are tall, posh buildings. That is the other side, the extreme the rich, that is the contrast. We don't value nature-we destroy and then we spend millions. We just don't value anything. There is extreme poverty one side and richness on the other side. We are responsible for all that. Then we spend a lot of money to conserve nature.

This remarkable dream brings together the issues of value and money associated with Oxygen. The division of the world into rich and poor is a primary aspect of psora, one which Hahnemann often refers to in his discussions on psora in *Chronic Diseases*. But the dream also highlights one more associated topic, that of consumption, or tuberculosis, which is an extension of psora – a poverty of oxygen. In the dream the fishes are gasping for oxygen in the form of air and water.

From the moment we are born, we consume oxygen in large quantities. Research studies indicate that the weight of oxygen we consume daily exceeds the total weight of the food consumed by us in the same time. This links the concept of consumption with TB, whereby we are unable to consume the air we need from the atmosphere, and as a concomitant we consume our living bodies. In the dream peoples' flesh is consumed and they are reduced to bones. One may therefore speculate that Oxygen is a tubercular remedy, as well as an anorexic one. Our constant sense of deficiency and dissatisfaction, due to the absence of our half-soul mate, is replaced by material need, and our primary material need is for Oxygen, a reflection of our ego's need for love, recognition and value.

Finally, the following Oxygen dream is reminiscent of our missing four-part soul, where we are left with two soul fragments, of which only the frontal one is conscious.

I am somewhere at a station and somebody is selling books. He was telling me that one book costs 10 rupees, outside it will cost more. I am telling that I will take 4 books for 40 rupees and the next time I will come I will buy more.

Oxygen gives us life, but, like the ego, oxygenation also sours and ages us. With the introduction of Oxygen into the human mix, we have gained ego and lost soul. The Oxygen ego binds with the Hydrogen soul to form the waters of our beings. Each one of us is now a water droplet, loosely connected through weak, ego-based electromagnetic bonds that hold the water molecules together and knit us into the relatively frail union of families and communities.

This newly acquired ego separates us from divine light. The Ozone firmament protects us from its intense rays.

Thus, the oxygen molecule both joins and separates the first and second periods. As O2, oxygen, it binds hydrogen into the waters of life. But its sister Ozone, O3, is the firmament between the fiery waters above (Hydrogen), and the waters below (oxygen). It is the firmament that separates ultimate truth from life on earth.

Now the earth was unformed and void, and darkness was upon the face of the deep; and the spirit of God hovered over the face of the waters.

Fluorine and neon

If oxygen creates water, and if ozone separates heavenly water from earthly water, what is the role of the two remaining elements in the period, fluorine and neon?

From the previous biblical analogy, we can assume that Day Two or 'Water Project A' terminates with ozone when the firmament is completed. Fluorine and neon therefore represent 'Water Project B', which occurs in the first half of the third day. Neon would thus correspond to the final stage which occurs when the waters have withdrawn to expose the earth ready for the birth of new life. This is confirmed by the proving symptoms and by several cases in this book, which express the feeling as 'At last I stand on the earth'.

From here on, the elements and salts of the third period represent the earth and its flora –: sodium, magnesium, aluminium, silicon, phosphorus

Water projects

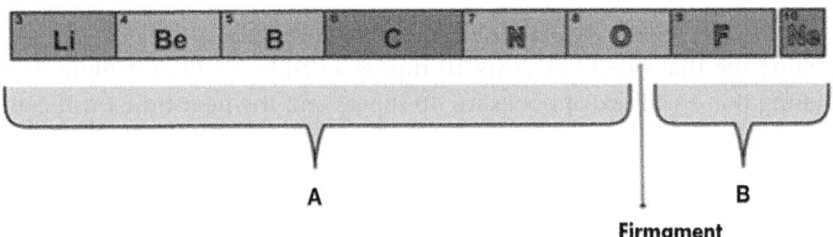

A

B

Firmament

Figure 14.9 The second period relating to Water Project A (Day Two) and Water Project B (first half of Day Three)

and sulphur. These elements combine with the organic elements of the second period to form life. Even deadly chlorine is an essential micronutrient for some plants. Argon completes the tree.

Before the earth can dry, the waters must withdraw. Fluorine therefore relates to the process by which the waters gather into one place.

And God said:

'Let the waters under the heaven be **gathered together unto one place**, and let the dry land appear.'

The strange thing about this verse is the *'one place'* factor. How can all the waters on earth be in one place? Rashi, a Jewish scholar, states that the 'one place' is referred to as *Oceania*, the great ocean, i.e. one great place. The Jewish canons of interpretation have lengthy discussions on the subject and this feat is generally considered a great miracle. Many examples are given of how 'a lot can be compressed into a little'.[19] One such example is that God's compression of water is analogous to the compression of a bunch of feathers by stepping on them.

There is only one element that has the awesome power to conquer and compress all the waters, and that is fluorine, the most chemically reactive and electronegative of all the elements. Its sudden, sometimes explosive, reaction can literally burn water as well as metals, glass, ceramics, carbon and bricks. It is so powerful that it can form compounds with rare gases, including xenon, radon, and krypton. In fact, it forms compounds with all the elements except neon and helium.

The extraordinary power of fluoride to combine with other elements also makes it the great separator. Just as it separates water from earth, it can wrench apart the two halves of our being. This is how it happens: Once the half-soul, composed of two soul gametes, is incarnated, one half is powerfully drawn forward towards the light of our eyes. In the beginning this seems like fun – finally a window to look out of. From the proving of Fluoric acid:

Pleasant sensation, as if the eyelids were wider opened, or the eyes more prominent, whereby the circle of the vision becomes more enlarged, the sight cleared, and he feels a kind of luxurious enjoyment while looking at the same things he is used to seeing every day.

The front half, one soul gamete and a quarter of the original soul, now forms our conscious identity, believing we live in our eyes, while the other half retreats to the shadows to form our subconscious. This separation, or splitting, is analogous to the separation of water from earth on the third day, as initiated by Fluorine and completed in Neon. Fluoric acid separates husband from wife, male from female, sex from love. From now on our alienated, two quarter-souls will yearn and seek each other, in the belief that a reunion will bring true love.

After the appearance of fluorine and the gathering of the waters, Neon completes Water Project B in the middle of the third day. At this point earth appears and, behold, the great division of earth and water is finished.

At last, I touch the earth.

I feel more stable now that my feet touch the earth while still having my head touching the heavens.

Neon ends the parting of earth and water, and we now move into the second part of Day Three, which corresponds with the first and last elements of the third period, sodium and chlorine. Natrum muriaticum, or common salt, symbolises the splitting of water and earth, and their intense desire for reunion, hence its dwelling by the seaside.

When the front and back quarters of our soul split, the psoric mirrors of our being trick us into believing that our missing quarter lives outside ourselves, that true love can be found in another person. Natrum muriaticum, which appears directly after the Neon split, is the first to fall for this illusion. Ultimately, its external love will be disappointed, unless it can be matched by an inner union.

Yet romance starts with 'sex on the beach', and from this liaison life will spring forth, in the form of seed, plant and child. The second part of the third day, and its corresponding third period, continue from the point where Neon finished, to develop the organic world of vegetation. In nature, this 'sex on the beach' is known as the water cycle. For this cycle to occur, we need the new dimension of height, which I will discuss in *Argon*.

In summary, the elements of the second period, up to and including oxygen, relate to the second day of creation. Carbon provides a womb in which oxygen captures hydrogen to create water. This second day is completed with ozone, which provides the firmament. O_3 or ozone, oxygen's triple-ego, is the black lie that both protects and separates organic life from the purity of spiritual light from above and splits the fiery waters of the first period from the oxygen-based waters below. Fluoride then contracts the waters into one place, hardening our ego into a one-sided identity. Neon breaks the waters, completing the process with our delivery onto an exposed earth, new life.

And it was good.

Cain and Abel

Another story that reflects the Neon concept is 'Cain and Abel', the first biblical account of murder. The two brothers quarrel because Abel's sacrifice is 'seen' and accepted by God, while Cain's is ignored. After Cain kills Abel he must become a fugitive and wander for the rest of his life. A mark is put on his forehead to protect him from the vagrancies of his predicament. The story concludes with the following warning:

> 'If you do what is right, will you not be accepted? But if you do not do what is right, **sin is crouching at your door**; it desires to have you, but you must master it.'

The Neon signatures of the brow chakra and of temptation knocking on the door echo in this story.

Adam and Eve are banished from the Garden of Eden, represented in the first period by Hydrogen and Helium. They then descend into the second earthly period, where they beget Cain and Abel.

Referring back to my Helium theory of soul evolution, Adam and Eve, combined as one person in their primary state, represent the complete four-part Helium soul. Once they 'see' each other naked they separate, which is analogous to both the soul splitting into two halves before incarnating into a material body and to their banishment from the Garden of Eden. Their children, Cain and Abel, represent the incarnated half-souls, and are subject to desire, the temptation at the door that we see in the Neon proving. It is this temptation that causes the half-soul to split into two quarter-souls. One quarter, represented by Abel, migrates forwards towards the light, at the eyes, so that God 'see's' his sacrifice. The second quarter, represented by Cain, the murderer, retreats to the shadowy recess of the subconscious. He is not seen.

From this time on, the conscious self is prone to battle with its shadow side. Temptation is always 'knocking on the door', enticing us with desires that our intellectual barrier, our firmament, does its best to ignore. Cain's mark on the brow chakra reminds us that the soul's real solution is to amalgamate the dark shadow side with the frontal 'light' aspects.

The Ten Commandments

In the previous book of this series[12] I related Moses to the remedies Hydrogen and Helium. The name Moses is derived from the word to 'pull out', or 'to withdraw', referring to the story of Moses being withdrawn from the waters of the Nile by the Pharaoh's daughter. In analogy we might say that she withdrew Moses, representing Hydrogen, from H_2O, leaving his Oxygen ego behind. Hence Moses is described in the Bible as the most modest person ever to walk the earth. Moses ascends the mountain where he meets and converses with the **one** God (Hydrogen), the only person in the Bible to meet God face to face. The mountain glows and quakes, and emits a great noise, the fusion of Hydrogen into Helium. Moses is given the **two** tablets (Helium) that contain the **Ten** Commandments (Neon).

These commandments serve two functions regarding our discussion of Neon. Firstly, they deal with the barrier of worship and respect between God and humanity, the firmament, i.e. *Thou shalt not take the name of the Lord thy God in vain*. Secondly, they create a boundary between humanity and its desires i.e. *Thou shalt not covet thy neighbour's house; thou shalt not covet thy neighbour's wife, nor his man-servant, nor his maid-servant, nor his ox, nor his ass, nor any thing that is thy neighbour's*. From Hydrogen to Helium to Neon: One into two into ten.

Ezekiel

Another biblical analogy is Ezekiel's vision of Yahweh's chariot in the book of *Ezekiel*, which mirrors the evolution of the soul from Helium to Neon. The narrative begins with the four faces of the heavenly creatures, which reflect the four-sided aspect of the soul described in *Helium*.[12] The vision of the wheels relates to the nature of the vital force as energy spinning at high speed that creates the gyroscopic forces to withstand gravity and keep life in vertical balance (more on this in the Krypton book of this series).

The following excerpt from *Ezekiel* describes these associations (the wording in bold refers to Helium symptoms and concepts):

> Now as I beheld the living creatures, behold one wheel at the bottom hard by the living creatures, at the four faces thereof. The appearance of the wheels and their work was like unto the colour of a beryl; and they **four had one likeness**; and their appearance and their work was as it were a **wheel within a wheel**. When they went, they went toward their **four sides**; they turned not when they went. As for their rings, they were high and they were dreadful; and **they four** had their rings **full of eyes round about**. And when the living creatures went, the wheels went hard by them; and when the living creatures were lifted up from the bottom, the wheels were lifted up. Whithersoever **the spirit** was to go, as the spirit was to go thither, so they went; and the wheels were lifted up beside them; **for the spirit of the living creature was in the wheels**.
>
> Ezekiel 1:15–20[20]

The description then moves to Neon's themes of two, of the great waters, of the firmament and of the split between upper and lower:

> And over the heads of the living creatures there was the likeness of **a firmament**, like the **colour of the terrible ice**, stretched forth over their heads above. And **under the firmament** were their wings conformable the one to the other; this one of them had **two which covered**, and that one of them had **two which covered, their bodies**. And when they went, I heard the noise of their wings like the noise **of great waters**, like the voice of the Almighty, a noise of tumult like the noise of a host; when they stood, they let down their wings. For, when there was a voice **above the firmament** that was over their heads, as they stood, they let down their wings. **And above the firmament** that was over their heads was the likeness of a throne, as the appearance of a **sapphire stone**; and upon the likeness of the throne was a likeness as the appearance of a man upon it above. And I saw as the **colour of electrum** [pale to bright yellow], as the appearance of fire round about enclosing it, from the appearance of his **loins and upward**; and from the appearance of his **loins and downward** I saw as it were the appearance of fire, and there was **brightness round about him**. As the appearance of the **rainbow that is in the cloud** in the day of rain, so was the appearance of the brightness round about.
>
> Ezekiel 1:22–28[20]

Cabbalistic connotations

The following section is relevant only for those who wish to investigate the relationship between the Cabbala and homoeopathic philosophy.

The Tree of Life is one of the basic models of the Cabbala.[i] It depicts the ten energetic centres called seffirot (spheres or seffira in the singular)

---

[i] Throughout the text I have spelt the word Cabbala in this way, although there are several different spellings for this word, each signifying different roots. In my opinion the initial letter C is more appropriate then K or Q, as it depicts the receptive, a womb-like image (Cabbala means to receive). The distinction between K and C will become clear in the study of Krypton.

through which God's light travels as it is attenuates from pure infinite spiritual light to a more terrestrial form of creation. Many other texts are available on this subject for the interested reader, so I will confine my discussion to Neon and the noble gases.

There are many correspondences between the cabbalistic Tree of Life and the noble gases. It must be made clear that this esoteric representation is not a fixed model, but rather a dynamic, fluid and interchangeable concept that encompasses many points of view. One cannot say that a particular noble gas corresponds uniquely to a specific seffira. Each of the ten seffirot encompass ideas from all the others and is thus a hologram of the whole. Thus, we may relate a particular aspect of a noble gas to one seffira in one model and to a different seffira in another.

The coloured line in Figure 14.10 depicts the passage of light as it descends from pure spirit to the material world. It is described in the Cabbala as a lightning bolt, moving not in a straight line but zigzagging down the tree. A direct light would be far too powerful, burning us with its truth. Each seffira is said to be of less intensity than the preceding one. A veil separates the consecutive emanations in their passage from spirit to matter. Hence the seffira Binah is one potency down from Chochma, or one step closer to terrestrial existence.

Keter, the first seffira, is the crown above our heads. It represents the infinite energy that precedes hydrogen, the universe just after the big bang but before the formation of the first atoms. Hydrogen and helium equate to the next seffira, Chochma, which means wisdom. Chochma is the initial spark of light that endows us with a holistic and unconstrained view of the whole.

Binah, the third seffira, denotes understanding or the realm of intellectual analysis. Binah transforms the ethereal wisdom of Chochma into analytical and logical thinking. It develops the cognitive faculty and articulates the holistic energy of Chochma into deductive understanding. This kind of intellectual analysis necessitates division; we separate conceptual ideas into components and compare this with that. Hence Binah begins with a split into two, the birth of mathematics and logic, and, as such, relates to Neon.

Judgement and reproach are prominent in the Neon proving which is why cabbalistic theology is useful to a deeper understanding of Neon. Binah is the first seffira of the left hand column. This column corresponds to judgement, a process that involves comparing, contrasting, preferring and deciding. The column of judgement is also associated with the female. While this may seem contrary to our common view of the loving mother, it is the female who must keep her feet on the earth so that she can make

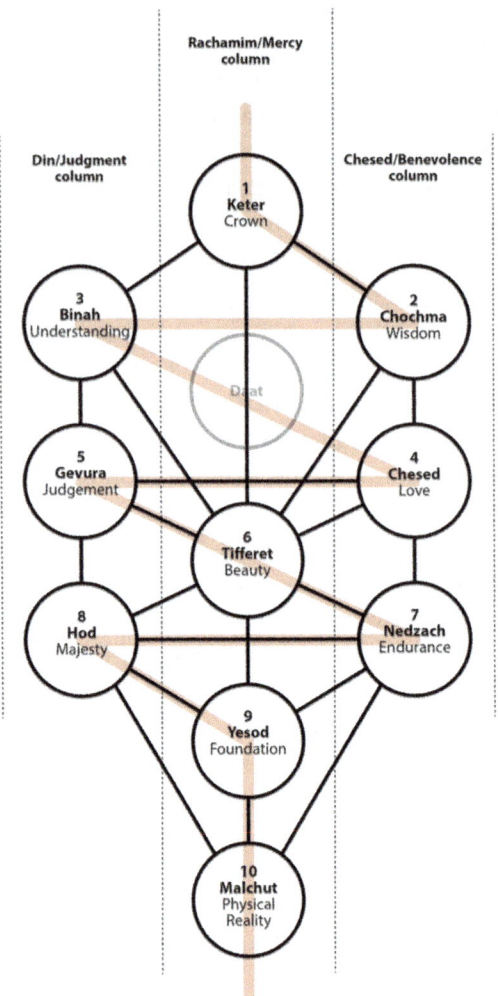

Figure 14.10 The Tree of Life

the tough and critical decisions of life: which single sperm to choose from the millions available, whom to marry, where to live, how to raise the kids.

By contrast, the right-hand column of Chesed (meaning benevolent acceptance) is connected with the male and represents an all encompassing, non-judgmental acceptance, as well as expansion of boundaries. Chesed is thus also connected with Helium, since male energy, like a helium balloon, may tend to float to the heavens unless it is tied down with some grounded common sense. Hence Binah is the ground to Chochma's spirituality. Remember, however, that this is not a simple male – female divide; each side contains the other.

The essence of Binah is said to be happiness, since happiness and joy result when insight from the undivided and ungraspable state of Chochma is transformed into the revealed state of Binah. However, the firmament, or the veil that separates Binah from Chochma,, will conceal the life-sustaining emanations from heaven unless we retain a window in the sky to access this divine energy.

The middle column, Rachamim, or Mercy, connects the crown with the seffirot of Daat, Tifferet, Yesod and Malchut. This is the vertical axis we encounter in Helium and Neon, but its influence can be felt only when we are 'aligned' with it. In cabbalistic writing, it is often referred to as 'Derech Hyashar' or the 'straight path'. This column represents the direct connection to heaven, the middle way.

The left path of Judgement, Din, represents immediate time or instant karma. If one transgresses, there is immediate retribution. The right path of Chesed, or Benevolence, perceives the world in the broadest and most lenient way possible. Like Helium, this line is not connected to the earthly passage of time. Our behaviour may deviate from the straight and narrow, but there is always time to make corrections, i.e. there is no immediate punishment; *'Never mind if I have another drink, tomorrow is another day.'* The middle path of Mercy gives us a limited amount of time to correct our transgressions. Hence Helium, on the right, does not connect to one's earthly deeds, whereas Neon, on the left, is ruled by time, desire, judgement and their consequences. The middle path may be found in Argon. We will wait and see.

Mishna and Zohar

The Mishna and Zohar are two Jewish canons of biblical interpretations. The following are some selected insights into the second day of creation, from these writings and from Jewish sages, including Maimonides and Rashi.[21]

- Water already existed on the first day. When God pronounced the second day, the middle layer of waters froze so that the top and bottom layers were separated. The firmament is frozen water (Maimonides).
- The Zohar states that the cold north wind froze the middle layer. This is the wind of Din, or judgment. (We learn that the quality of cold judgment enters life in Neon-JS). The waters above were separated from the waters below by tears.

- The waters were split exactly in the middle so that top and bottom layers are exactly equal in depth. This creates a factor of two.
- There is an empty space between the top waters and the firmament and between the bottom waters and the firmament.
- The firmament is about three fingers wide, and resembles a tray.
- Why is there no pronouncement on the second day: *'And God saw that it was good'* as there is on all the other days of creation? Because on the second day, hell was created as division and conflict came into being.
- The Bible does not say *'it was good'* on the second day because the creation of water is not completed until the third day when water separates from land, after which God pronounces it 'good'.
- The division is not merely a barrier but a change of form between upper and lower waters, just like the differentiation between light and dark. Water has three forms, gas, liquid, solid, like our spiritual states, higher, lower and pure material (Maimonides).
- There are three types of water: below the firmament – the rivers and seas, the firmament itself and the water over the firmament (Maimonides).

The word firmament is 'rakia' in Hebrew, from the same root as 'ikar' or 'principles'. Hence the firmament is a set of principles, which set apart the purely spiritual, undivided world above from the logical world below.

Said Rabbi Isaac: 'In the human body, there exists an organ called the diaphragm, separating the heart from the abdomen, so that what the former receives or takes in is transmitted to the latter. So is it with the firmament in the midst of the waters, or the higher and lower spheres of existence. What it receives from the higher it transmits to the lower spheres for the maintenance and continuity of human and annual life. There is an allusion to this in the words, 'And the veil shall divide between the holy place and the holy of Holies'' (Zohar).

- The Zohar states: The firmament is a 'locked garden' (a reference to King Solomon's *'Song of Songs'*). This locked garden is the barrier between male and female principles.

Don't say water-water

The following is the story of four sages and their search for enlightenment. What seems like a simple walk in the garden becomes quite complex with a deeper look. It can be understood as an attempt by the four-part soul to penetrate the Neon firmament so as to reunite with God in Hydrogen.

Well-known in the Talmud and repeated in the Cabbala, the story tells of four sages who enter a secret garden known as 'Pardes' (paradise or orchard), an analogy for a mystical voyage through the different levels of consciousness and cosmic experience. The word 'Pardes' is also an acronym for the four levels of perception which are:

1. The simple and basic meaning as read.
2. Hints to a hidden meaning, first interpretation.
3. The deeper search or inquiry.
4. The highest level, that of the mystic secret.

The four sages set out on the journey through the four levels of Pardes, seeking the highest level of realisation and spirituality by means of biblical study, meditation and exercises in personal potentisation. On this quest one of the four sages dies, one goes insane and one becomes a heretic. Only the fourth arrives at the source of mystical secrets and makes it back safely. What interests us in relation to Neon is the warning they receive before setting out. Here is the story:

> The Rabbis taught: Four sages entered the Pardes [literally 'the orchard.'] They ascended to heaven by utilising the Divine Name, i.e., they achieved a spiritual elevation through intense meditation on God's Name. They were Ben Azzai, Ben Zoma, Elisha ben Avuya, and Rabbi Akiva. Rabbi Akiva said to them [prior to their ascension]: 'When you come to the place of pure marble stones, do not say, 'Water – Water!' for it is said, 'He who speaks untruths shall not stand before my eyes''. Ben Azzai gazed [at the Divine Presence] and died. Ben Zoma gazed and lost his sanity. Elisha ben Avuya became a heretic. Rabbi Akiva entered in peace and left in peace.
>
> On hearing this story, the ancient Saba [grandfather, old man, sage-JS] stood up and said to his teacher Rabbi Shimon bar Yochai: 'Rabbi, Rabbi! What is the meaning of what Rabbi Akiva said to his students, 'When you come to the place of pure marble stones, do not say 'Water – Water!' lest you place yourselves in danger, for it is said, 'He who speaks untruths shall not stand before My eyes.' But it is written, 'There shall be a firmament between the waters and it shall separate between water above the firmament and water below the firmament.' Since the Torah describes the division of the waters into upper and lower, why should it be problematic to mention this division?
>
> Rabbi Shimon bar Yochai replied, 'Saba, it is proper that you reveal this secret that the circle of disciples has not grasped clearly.'
>
> The ancient Saba answered, 'Rabbi, Rabbi. Surely the pure marble stones are the letter yud – one the upper yud of the letter aleph, and one the lower yud of the letter aleph.'[22]

There follows a lengthy and complex cabbalistic explanation of this quandary, which can be read in the source material. Here I will add my own insights, based on the Neon proving, which differ slightly from the original interpretation. My perception is partly based on the intrinsic meaning of the letters in key words and on the numerical values attributed to Hebrew letters.

First let us look at the spelling and meaning of the words and letters. The word 'water' (*mayim*) in Hebrew, מים, and the word 'marble' (*shayish*), שיש, look similar in Hebrew. Both are composed of the middle letter Yud (or Yod) surrounded either by two Mem's (מ) or two Shin's (ש), thus being easily interchanged and confused. Both are palindromes, which makes it difficult to know if you are coming or going. From the story, we learn that marble is the place where the separation between water and water occurs. Hence in this analogy, marble represents the firmament.

In the biblical story of creation the upper waters are called *shamayim* meaning sky or heaven. The word *sha-mayim* in Hebrew is composed of the letter *Shin* plus the word 'water': שמים. Hence the word *sha-mayim* is composed of the letters of the word 'marble' (ש), plus the word 'water', literally meaning *the waters of heaven which are beyond marble*. The letter *Shin* also represents fire, hence heaven is known as 'fire-water'. This represents the first period of the periodic table (upper waters or hydro-gen).

In the first part of the story, the four sages can be compared to the four parts of the soul. Their journey ascending to the Divine Presence takes them up the periodic table towards Helium, Hydrogen and Heaven. They must pass through the window in the firmament to transcend the material second period to reach the spiritual first period.

Dream: Waiting for the lift (also waiting for the light) to the sixth or seventh floor to meet Our Father. (Helium proving)

The sages arrive at the firmament, which separates the first and second periods and the two levels of water. This firmament looks like shimmering marble, which can in fact resemble water. But it is a deception, a material diversion from the true journey. (The proving of Marble depicts attractive external beauty combined with self-centred decadence). The sages should not acknowledge this false firmament by saying 'water-water'. To pass through the firmament into the first period, they must be noble and truthful, for it is said, '*He who speaks untruths shall not stand before my eyes.*' Any sage who is not completely upright will be deceived by the marble of desire and will be unable to pass through. Only Rabbi Akiva passes the test and ascends to the first period unharmed.

The story offers no reason why the old sage chooses Aleph (Figure 14.11) of all the letters as a solution to the problem. Aleph is the first letter of the Hebrew alphabet (the word Alphabet is literally derived from the Hebrew Aleph-Bet). It is my understanding that Aleph, which is traditionally

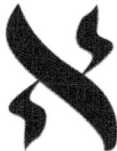

Figure 14.11 Aleph

assigned the number one, represents hydrogen and the first period. (Bet, the second letter, is the first letter of the Bible in the word *Bereshit* or *Beginning*, representing the Big Bang and the second element, helium).

The old man refers to the graphic shape or image of the letter Aleph, a frequent practice in cabbalistic thinking, as one letter is often composed of several others. This is how the Hebrew letters which create 'Aleph' look (Figure 14.12).

Aleph is composed of an upright Yud at the top right and an upside-down Yud at the bottom left, separated by a Vav; the diagonal line between them. Vav literally means hook, which both connects things and separates them. It is the vertical line connecting above and below, but also the firmament. The old man is indicating that Aleph depicts the separation between the upright Yud above, heavenly waters, and the upside down Yud below, the lower waters. Thus the lower waters are a mirror image of the upper waters. As we have seen, the second period signifies living through a mirror in a world of deception.

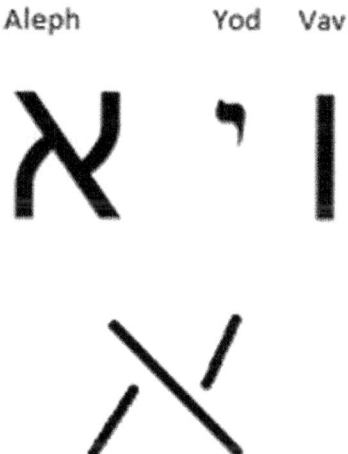

Figure 14.12 *The Hebrew letter Aleph, composed of a Vav and two Yud's, one above and one below*

In Hebrew numerology the letter Yud, the 10th letter of the alphabet, is equivalent to the number 10. Ten is the number of electrons in the water molecule as well as in the neon atom. QED.

The word *mayim*, water, is composed of the letters Mem-Yud-Mem, which have the corresponding numerical value of 40, 10, 40, giving a sum of 90. This is the numerical equivalent to the word *tsadik*, meaning righteous or noble person. Only a Noble person, such as the fourth sage Rabbi Akiva, can differentiate the two waters and transcend the firmament that separates them.

Tsadik and *Klipa*, the light and its shell

> The noble, upright, truthful physician works in the night; he works in the dark; he works quietly; he is not seeking for praise.
>
> JT Kent[23]

In Jewish theology the concept of 'tsadik' refers to the 'righteous one', which is usually a Biblical figure or spiritual master. To understand *tsadik*, the noble person, in cabbalistic terms, we must first learn about the concept of klipa, which the tsadik must encounter and penetrate.

The Cabbala introduces the concept of klipa (Klipot in pleural), which means peel, shell or covering, similar to the peel of a fruit. Different cabbalistic traditions have a variety of complex interpretations of the klipa, so I will simplify it into one common denominator for the purpose of this discussion. The following is my own attempt to weave together several concepts, and hence these thoughts belong to no one, particular tradition.

The klipa is a dark layer or shell whose purpose is to shield or hide the light, but at the same time to protect it. It wraps around the sparks or fragments of creation, concealing their light. The klipa can be understood as evil, hiding our inner light, or beneficial, protecting us from too much light when we are not ready for it, when our vessel is not strong enough to receive the full light of God. Klipot are a direct opposite to God's light, as they are composed from a 'desire to receive' while God's light is pure 'desire to give'. This 'desire to receive', or selfish egotism, differentiates us from the all-giving light of God. It is said that souls incarnate as a result of God bestowing light with a quality of selfishness. This relates to our understanding of Helium, the pure soul, and the concept of the firmament represents the quality of selfishness.

While one may think of these shells as originating from the dark side, they also have a positive side. Just as the peel protects a fruit until it is ripe, so these dark shells protect us and help show us that desire for the super-ficial, or anything other than unification with universal light, can only end with discontent. They are teachers, a 'help against us', and through beating ourselves against them again and again, we may learn how to rectify our lives.

The firmament may represent the first, or one of the first, Klipot (shells). One level down from the light of the first day, the firmament shields and separates the fire-water heavens above from the watery seas below (the names of three of the major Klipot are 'stormy wind', 'the great cloud', and 'the all-consuming fire').

In our periodic table analogy, one of the manifestations of the firmament is the ozone layer, a dark layer that both conceals and protect us from the UniVersal light of truth. It is a layer of comforting lies, of intellectual wrangulations and logical computations, a layer that keeps us locked in 'desire to receive', the discontent so prominent in Neon. (use this format)

Neon has two ways to escape this ozone shell or klipa. It can prostrate itself into the worldly cycle of desire and discontent, the 'itch-scratchy' show. In this mode it will have to crawl back along the second period, holding its breath as it sneaks past the ozone barrier in the search of a Carbon diamond or Lithium medication.

Alternatively Neon can rectify itself by becoming upright, perpendicu-larly penetrating the narrow 'window of the sky' directly above, plugging into the universal source of energy, light and love, at which time it becomes a *tsadik*.

The Cabbala contains the tradition of *tsadik*, or righteous, enlightened person. The *tsadik* has rectified his life through good deeds (unselfish giving for no physical or spiritual reward). Thus, he/she is connected to the light. He penetrates the ozone layer by being upright – physically, morally and spiritually. According to legend, at all times there are 36 such righteous people in the world. We can interpret 36 to represent Krypton (atomic number 36) and a double Argon (atomic number 18). We can see the vertical, noble line of the *tsadik* stretching directly upwards through Helium to the source of sources.

The Hebrew word *tsadik* (from the root 'justice') represents this righteous person. It is also a letter with the value of 90 in Hebrew numerology (Figure 14.13), which is considered highly significant in esoteric terms. We could relate this to 90° or a line perpendicular to the earth.

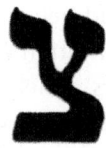

Figure 14.13 *The Hebrew letter 'tsadik'*

There are four Hebrew letters in the full word *tsadik*, the enlightened one:

צדיק

- צ   *Tsadik* – represents the upright or an angle of 90°
- ד   *Dalet* – means window or door
- י   *Yod* – Represents God and the number 10 – the Ten Commandments. (Only the tip of the *Yod* represents the infinite light)
- ק   *Kof* – has two meanings: the higher meaning represents holiness, the lower is an imitating monkey. *Kof* means 'monkey', 'to copy'. It is also the first letter of *klipa*. It is the only regular letter whose shape extends downwards below the line. It can pull us down.

To summarise this alphabetical analogy, an upright, righteous person can penetrate the window of the sky and reach God to become holy or can tilt and remain a monkey, i.e. not fulfilling our full human potential. Only thirty-six out of seven billion people will make it. The rest of us will continue to strive towards it.

Neon entices us with its selfish desire to receive, and thus we are trapped in the earthly world of discontent, like babies ruled by desire who are desperately grasping at any substitute for their mother, herself a pale substitute for the sea of souls.

Ultimately, Neon can teach us to become upright, to break through our inner firmament and touch the light.

In which case we will glow.

References

1 http://www.math.brown.edu/~banchoff/gc/Flatland/
2 Flammarion C. *L'atmosphère: météorologie populaire* Paris: Libraire Hachett et Cie, 1888.
3 http://en.wikipedia.org/wiki/Titan_%28mythology%29
4 http://en.wikipedia.org/wiki/Titan_%28moon%29
5 http://en.wikipedia.org/wiki/Titanium
6 http://www.enchantedlearning.com/subjects/astronomy/planets/uranus/
7 http://www.astrologyzone.com/tools/uranus.html
8 http://www.world-nuclear.org/info/Nuclear-Fuel-Cycle/Introduction/What-is-Uranium–How-Does-it-Work-/#.UhVPhX-9yPQ.
9 http://en.wikipedia.org/wiki/Seven-league_boots
10 http://www.universetoday.com/18955/tilt-of-uranus/
11 http://www.universetoday.com/73222/what-is-a-quasar/
12 Sherr J. *Dynamic Materia Medica: Helium*. Glasgow: Saltire Books, 2013.
13 Midrash Rabbah, B'reshith Rabbah.
14 Stratospheric Ozone http://www.ozonelayer.noaa.gov/science/basics.htm.
15 Schadde A. *Ozone*. Washington DC: Alethea Book Company, 1997.
16 Dr Chetna N. Shukla E-mail: drchetna@123india.com
17 A song by the British band *Sweet*, co-written by guitarist Andy Scott and Trevor Griffin.
18 Individual proving of Oxygen by Camilla Sherr.
19 Midrash Rabbah, B'reshith Rabbah, Zohar.
20 http://www2.trincoll.edu/~kiener/RELG109_Ezk1.html
21 Midrash Rabbah, B'reshith Rabbah, Zohar.
22 Edited and abbreviated from several Talmudic texts. One of these references is *The Talmud*. (Chagiga 14b), Zohar (I, 26b) and Tikunei Zohar (Tikun 40) report the following incident regarding four Mishnaic Sages http://ascentofsafed.com/cgi-bin/ascent.cgi?Name=pardes
23 Kent JT. *Lectures on Homeopathic Materia Medica*. Philadelphia PA: Boericke & Tafel, 1905. p. 3. Also: New Delhi: B. Jain Publications, 2010.

15

FURTHER ANALOGIES

The four elements

So far we have concentrated on Neon's affinity to water. However, using the model of the circle of four elements, in which Water and Earth are polarities on an axis, we understand that Neon's water affinity must necessarily have a balancing affinity with the opposite polarity of Earth.[1] Neon represents a split of tension along the horizontal line of Earth and Water. This split is apparent in water project B, the separation of earth and water in the first half of the third day of creation. We can imagine this horizontal line as the firmament that separates Fire above from Air below (Figure 15.1).

Earth represents dryness. Earth-related symptoms, such as dryness of the mouth, nose, throat, respiration, stool, skin and mucous membranes, are prominent in the proving of Neon, and correlate with Earth. Neon also has

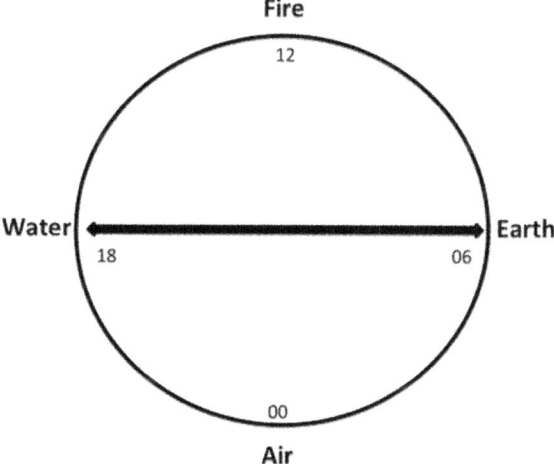

Figure 15.1 Circle of four elements, with times of the day. Neon is on the Earth – Water axis

an afternoon – evening aggravation, at 15–20 hours, 18 hours and 20–21 hours, which correlates with the Earth-related times on the circles (Figure 15.1).

This Earth aspect of Neon also appears in the following mental expressions:

At last, I touch the earth.

I feel more stable now that my feet touch the earth while my head still touches the heavens.

This relationship to Earth is illustrated in Case 12:7, '*I have arrived in the sphere of the earth,*' and in the follow-up of Case 12:13:

Two days after the remedy all of a sudden I felt the earth! Before the earth was puzzling me with her gravity. Now I feel like being in the womb of the mother again, but the universal mother.

In view of the symptoms and case expressions above, we can see that the Neon soul has now finally manifested as a new baby incarnating onto the Earth. This evolution can be seen in the following illustration, in which I have combined the circle of four elements with a spiral image of the periodic table (Figure 15.2). In this diagram I compare the elements (remedies), and their cosmological analogies. Also included are the stages of soul incarnation and the corresponding stages of pregnancy.

Figure 15.2 represents the four elements and the four points between the elements. These intermediate points are Air-Water, which is a static energy (cold and wet-ice); Water-Fire, which is expansive (wet and hot-steam); Fire-Earth, which is dynamic (hot and dry) and finally Earth-Air, which is contractive (dry and cold, metal). This is the standard four element configuration as is well known in some homoeopathic circles. Onto this I have superimposed the elements of the first two periods (in circles), the evolution of the soul (blue italics) and stages of pregnancy (in green). The correspondences are quite instructive. We will be comparing the circle of four elements to the evolution of the periodic table, pregnancy and soul incarnation.

Begin at the top of the diagram and move clockwise. Fire corresponds to the singularity and to the Big Bang – all souls are one. This is also the point of orgasm before conception. Once Hydrogen forms there is a separation from God that marks the beginning of the formation of an individual soul. Four Hydrogen nuclei, or soul gametes fuse into an individual Helium soul at the point of maximum expansion. (See *Helium*[1] for a full explanation). This corresponds to the point of conception, after which the embryonic cells start multiplying.

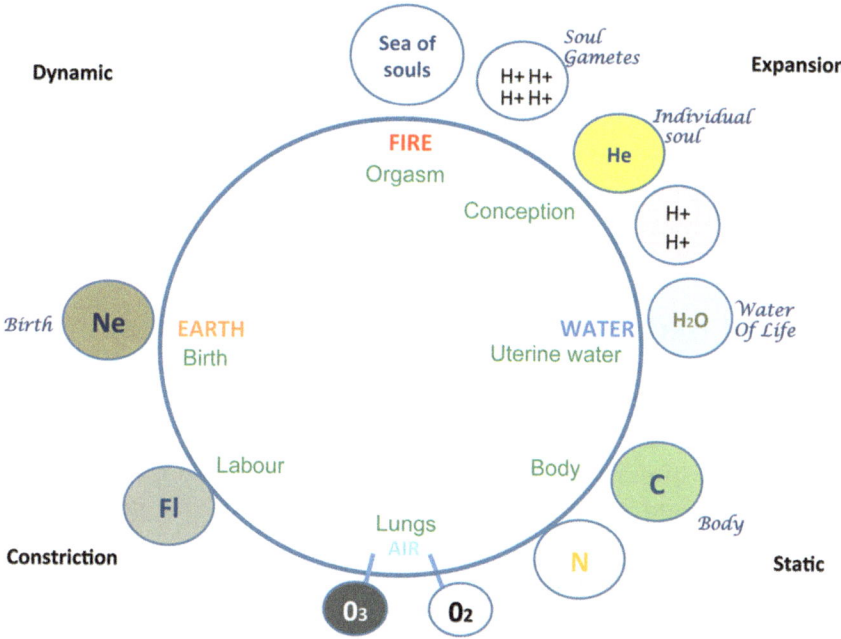

Figure 15.2 *The periodic spiral that depicts soul evolution and the four elements*

The full soul now splits into two halves or soul mates, which incarnate as two hydrogen ions and combine with oxygen to form the Water of Life. This is directly opposite neon, on the Water–Earth axis. Likewise, during pregnancy the uterus fills with water.

Carbon and nitrogen then form, creating physical structure and barriers respectively, while aligning with the point of maximum static, the material body.

Oxygen and Ozone naturally appear at the Air point, Oxygen on the white/life side and Ozone on the black/death side. At the corresponding time, towards the end of pregnancy, the fetal lungs develop. Fluoride then follows, with the highest electronegativity and reactivity of the periodic table – the ability to attract all other elements – and thus represents maximum contraction. This is analogous to the contraction of the waters into one place in Day Three, as well as the breaking of waters just before birth. Once the earth is exposed, the newborn Neon finally touches the earth.

We will continue to spiral this diagram into the next book in this series, *Argon*, beginning with Natrum muriaticum, the first and last elements of the third period, representing salt and sea, the Earth-Water axis.

Window of the Sky

In acupuncture there are certain points called 'Window of the Sky', which, according to some modern acupuncturists, connect our Spiritual Self to our Physical Self. Most of these points are located around the neck. They provide a way to access that which lies hidden in the spiritual world.

There is also a U2 song called *'Window in the Skies'*.

Biblical Neon superheroes

Each noble gas can be associated with one or more superheroes. Previously, I mentioned Noah as the superhero of Neon, who saves the continuity of living things through his upright righteousness. For over a year Noah lives in a water world, water above and water below. The Bible says that the windows of the skies literally opened for Noah.

In Noah's story the Neon theme of two-ness becomes apparent in the choice of pairs of animals. God's covenant with Noah is symbolised by the Neon rainbow in the sky. The end of the story moves to the third period of the periodic table, with the number three and all its associations. Noah has three sons who spawn all the people in the world. The next generation attempt to move into the third dimension of geometry and height by building the tall tower of Babel, perhaps because of the trauma of the flood, but this attempt is doomed to failure – they remain in the second dimension.

Another biblical analogy to Neon is the story of King Solomon, whose Hebrew name is Shlomo, meaning both wholeness and peace. He is the wisest of men, a spiritual teacher. One of Solomon's most well-known sayings is, 'There is nothing new under the sun',[2] a perfect representation of Neon, the 'new' element, which sits under the Helium sun. Solomon builds the temple, the physical structure to house God's spirit. His soul mate is the Queen of Sheba. The Queen of Sheba is mentioned several times in the Oncorhynchus or Salmon proving, and this remedy matches her long journey to find a soul mate. From clinical experience I have found Oncorhynchus to be a complementary remedy to Neon. Yet, like a true Neon, King Solomon succumbs to the itch of his desires, women being his main weakness, and he keeps a thousand wives.

There are also several analogies between Jesus and Neon. (Words in bold indicate Neon concepts.) Jesus, a young, radical Jewish rabbi living in Israel, was a spiritual teacher who heralded a **new age**, the age of **Pisces and water**. According to Christian theology, the nativity of Jesus represents the

incarnation of God in human form, **free of sin** and acting in obedience to
the divine will of God. Jesus is able to undo the damage caused by the fall
of the first man, Adam, and create an opportunity for salvation, offering a
passage between the second period and Hydrogen's 'Kingdom of Heaven'.
Jesus **preached love, acceptance and gratitude**. Much of the legend
around his nativity focuses on the birth of a new child to the Virgin Mary,
and a complete, single soul that gives rise to new life, i.e Helium to Neon.
The Three Kings follow the **star** to find Jesus. Christians believe in the
'**second coming**'.

I have lost the delusion, which I have always had, that I could walk on
water.
Dream of being a successful spiritual teacher.
Dream of being in a crowd with a spiritual teacher.
I now feel forgiven for the ultimate sin.
Overwhelming sensation of being surrounded by love.
Before I just wanted enlightenment, but now I am aware that there are
higher states of consciousness. I have set my sights higher.

'And the two shall become one flesh; so they are no longer two, but one flesh'.
Mark 10:8[3]

Behold, I stand at the door and Knock: if any man hear my voice, and open the
door, I will come in to him, and sup with him, and he with me.'
Revelations 3:20[4]

Alchemical stage – Dissolution

Dissolution, the second alchemical stage, neatly compares to Neon's watery
and child-based energies. In the previous book of this series, I related the
seven noble gases to the seven alchemical stages and compared Helium to
the first stage of Calcination, the fire of transformation that reduces a
substance to ashes. On the personal alchemical journey, the fire of Calcifi-
cation softens and prepares the ego for transformation, but the personality
needs to be processed further by Dissolution.

Dissolution happens once the ashes of Calcination are dissolved in water.
Water has the power to erode and corrode metals, so that Dissolution is
sometimes represented by rust. Emotionally, the dissolving of old and stuck
emotions is often experienced as tears, crying and sobbing.

Dissolution of the ego is not easy but is essential for liberation of the
true self. Those with strong personalities and well-defended egos may have
more difficulty dissolving their barriers. If we can burn the ego's barriers in

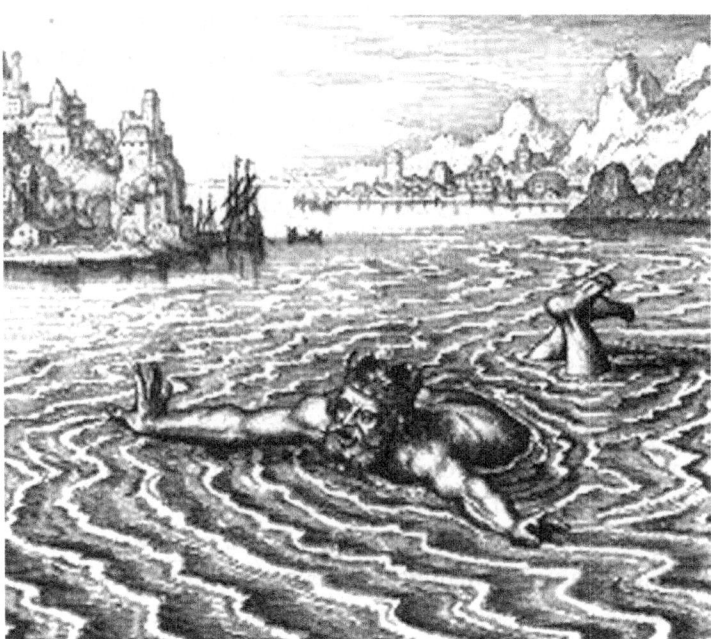

Figure 15.3 Dissolution

calcinations and dissolve the emotions that remain, we will be able to take responsibility for our own issues, instead of unconsciously projecting them onto others and experiencing them as external problems. Our demanding Neon baby can use its water to mature and develop new dimensions.

From an alchemical point of view Dissolution involves a melting of the ego, as in the process of openly weeping. Many of our early emotional experiences are suppressed and held in abeyance. If we can melt dry and authoritarian mental control, repressed and painful emotions will float to the surface. By allowing these emotions to be expressed we are able to bring them to our full consciousness and dissolve past issues. This may result in a flow of energy, leading to a feeling of bliss. On the other hand, if we choose to ignore these issues and distract ourselves with anything from drugs to television, the hard knots of the past will just coagulate further.

Sometimes accidents or illnesses force the process of Dissolution upon us, but from such misfortunes growth and maturation may occur.

Within our bodies, Dissolution can be felt as a Kundulini rising, the opening of energy channels, which cleanse and recharge every cell of our being. On the planetary level Dissolution can be seen as a purification, a clearing out of old structures and impurities, just as the Great Flood destroyed the old sinful generation and liberated the righteous.[5]

Lotus

In Silvie's second proving of Neon there are several references to the lotus flower.

Picture of lotus in my head.
Dreams of lotus stems – muddy and surrounded by water.
Felt I was a lotus just about to open – the water gets deeper, the wind ripples the surface.

In the realm of potency, kingdoms do not form a rigid grid of mineral, animal or plant remedies; analogies often extend cross-kingdom. It is therefore interesting to examine Lotus in search for possible correspondences to Neon.

The lotus is a beautiful flower to behold, with a strong relationship to water. An aquatic perennial, the lotus's roots dig into the muddy soil of a river or pond, while the pure white or pink flower floats above the surface. The lotus is unique in that it flowers and fruits at the same time.

The lotus features in many myths and bears a strong relationship to spirituality. Because its flower rises from the water at dawn and closes and sinks at night, the ancient Egyptians considered the lotus to represent the sun, creation and rebirth. They believed that the universe was created at Heliopolis when a lotus flower arose out of a primeval being named Nun

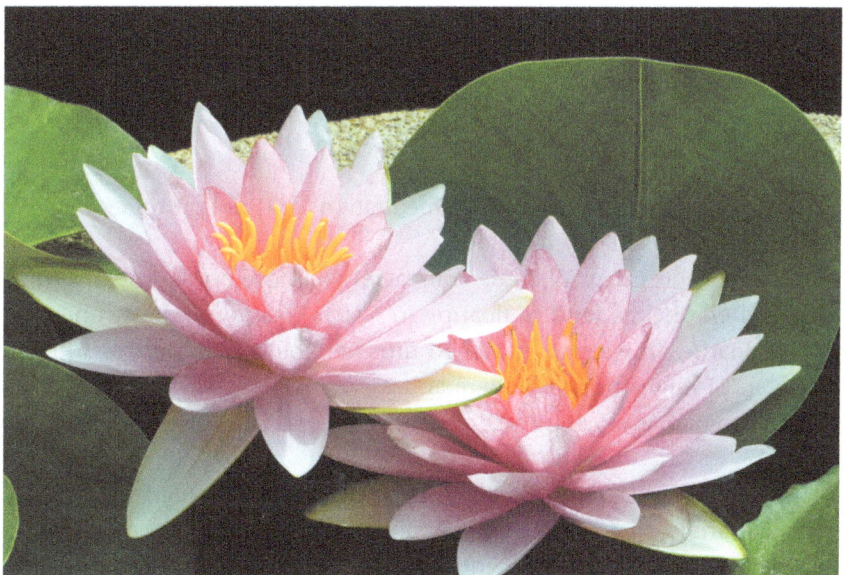

Figure 15.4 *Lotus flower*

(Neon?), who was an unending sea of still and lifeless water. Along with the lotus flower came a hill of dry land. This is reminiscent of Neon's relationship to the separation of water and Earth at the end of the biblical water project in Day Three. The Egyptians also used the symbol of one lotus flower for the number 1,000 and two lotus flowers for the number 2,000.

Buddhism also attributes important symbolism to the lotus flower. Buddhists regard the flower's ability to bloom far above its muddy roots as a metaphor for freeing oneself from the troubles of life and transcending the pain of human existence. The Buddha says 'In this way the human heart doesn't give rise to evil desires or evil thoughts. It's like the blue, red and white lotuses that grow in the water but bear no water.'[6]

The symbols of pollution and purity surrounding the lotus are important to practitioners of Mahayana Buddhism. Just as the root and flower of the lotus merge into one, so there is no distinction between pollution and purity. The Bodhisattva embraces purity of thoughts and actions, believing that dichotomies do not exist – 'muck is luck, evil is good, pollution is purity'. Therefore, the lotus ''doesn't grow in the highlands but rather it blooms in the vile swamps'.[7]

The stalk of the lotus flower, which grows long and pushes the flower above the water's surface, is extremely flexible. Because of its tough fibres, the stem is resistant to breaking, but can easily bend. This quality has been used in poetry to represent strong family or romantic relationships that are not diminished by distance because they are connected at the heart.[5]

We see several of these lotus themes mirrored in the Neon proving. Pure water and dirty mud, one and two, birth and rebirth, bliss and enlightenment, desire and dependency, flower in the mud. The following symptoms from the proving of the Sacred Lotus (Nelumbo nuciferea) illustrate the relationship between Lotus themes and Neon:[8]

Floating feeling: . . . I went into meditation. And as I sat there, I felt like I was floating, like I was a balloon.

. . . I had this image of those compasses you have on dashboards sometimes where they're kind of floating in water. Like my mind was here but it was floating in water and I could turn here but my mind was still over there and I might turn over here and it was over there. It was like it was never in synch, everything was always floating in this little thing I call my head.

Altered states: Dream: Working on house. There is a small square tower with a shingle on top that another individual is trying to complete and may abuse the power of it. By entering, can pass between times – into other times and/or dimensions.

Disconnection: . . . I didn't feel really connected with people. Like I felt like I couldn't make a strong connection with them, and didn't.

Vertigo: Only thing today was a jittery dizziness as I was squatting to finish some concrete – perhaps it was the fluorescent lights. . . .

Movies

In the 2012 movie *Life of Pi,* Max Cohen is a mathematical genius. Since he looked too long at the sun as a child, he is locked in the Neon world of numbers, patterns and headaches, separated from the spiritual first period (Helium-Hydrogen) and out of touch with the third emotional period, (Argon, Natrum muriaticum and friends). His door stays locked to the outside world; he is oblivious to the constant knocking. A cabbalist tries to use him to discover the mathematical code for the name of God, symbolising the ascent into the first spiritual period. Meanwhile Max constantly fights off the gooey world of emotions, sex, insects and the stock market beckoning from the third period below (to be explained in the Argon book). He is suspended between heaven and earth, Helium and Argon, in his Neon number prison. Like his ancestor, one of the four sages who tried to penetrate the firmament from the second period into the first, Max is going insane. His friend Sol (Sun) cannot save him. Eventually Max is given the code, the secret name of God expressed in a mathematical number. But the knocking on his door and mind continues, and Max is going insane. He finally answers the knocking by drilling a hole into his head and destroying his brain. With a newfound peace, he ascends into the world of Hydrogen and Helium, the sun.

The Matrix (1999), a science fiction action movie, is also highly illustrative of Neon. Neo, a young man living a purposeless, drugged-out life is summoned by a group of Jedi-like rebels with the words 'Knock-knock Neo'. He is given a choice between a blue pill and a red pill – to see the truth or continue living a lie. Neo chooses truth, and therefore gets to see beyond the firmament, in this case the 'matrix'. A mathematical software grid that projects a false reality over a sick world, the matrix hides the true state of humanity. The truth is that people have been taken over by an unknown force and are imprisoned as foetuses under the sea. They are used to generate the power that keeps the delusion going. As Neo gets closer to knowing the truth he becomes taller and more upright, both physically and morally, and consequently more and more powerful, performing super-human feats. Neo has stepped through the window in the sky to a place beyond the matrix and he is now known to be the 'One'. His accomplice,

Trinity, is his connection to the material world, thus uniting the first, second and third periods. Neo transcends to the first period of boundless possibilities, but the rest of the world chooses to stay behind and live the delusion.

Waterworld (1995), a big-budget flop of a movie, is about a post-apocalyptic flood. There is no land to be seen anywhere, and Kevin Costner and his merry band of men survive on boats. Water, water everywhere and no earth to be seen.

Lou Klein has drawn my attention to *Rain Man* (1988) as a good analogy to Neon. In this movie, Dustin Hoffman plays an idiot savant, an autistic and maths genius. It is this mathematical layer of intellect that seems to separate him from the world.

Poems that represent aspects of Neon

The Sound of Silence
Song lyric by Paul Simon[9]

And the people bowed and prayed
To the neon god they made
And the sign flashed out its warning
In the words that it was forming
And the sign said the words of the prophets

Are written on the subway walls
And tenement halls
And whispered in the sounds of silence

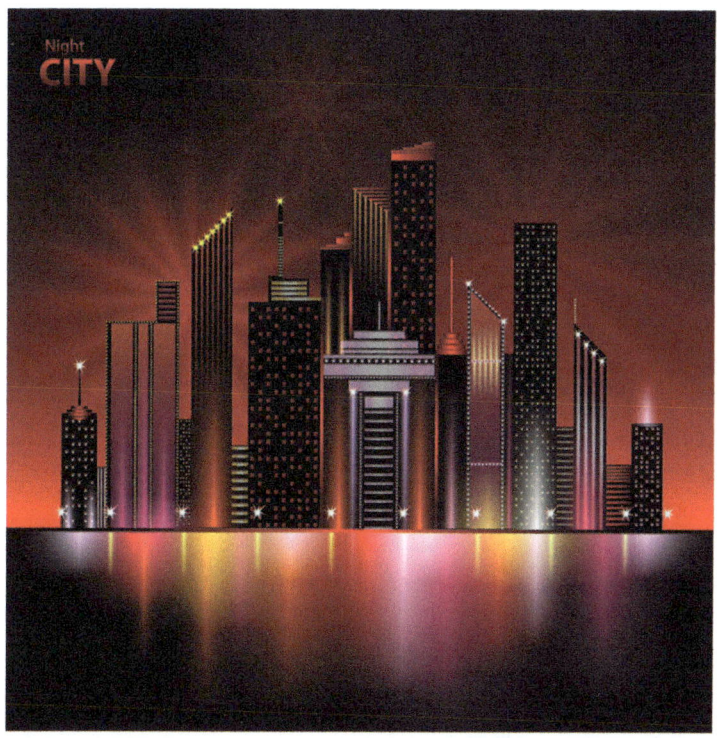

Figure.15.5 *Neon City*

Neon[10]

By Nathan Long

You're not so bright,
hanging out in a bar
all hours of the day–
like no one has ever
thought of that before!
Like there's something
noble in losing yourself
in glass after glass after
glass. Listen, buddy,
at least make yourself
useful: do you got a light?
And don't tell me you've
got something important
to say; there's never any –
thing new under the sun.

Neon lights[10]

By Heather A. Young

Illuminating cities of sin,
shamelessly calling out
to deviant children
of wonderfully dark indulgences.
Painting red, the faces
of Las Vegas street walkers.
Painting blue, the naked bodies
of New York's dancers.
Giving a gritty underworld
a vibrant, glamorous light
in which to thrive.
Its gentle electric hum
a breathing pulse,
festering in the midst of
concrete and steel.
A satire on organic chemistry.

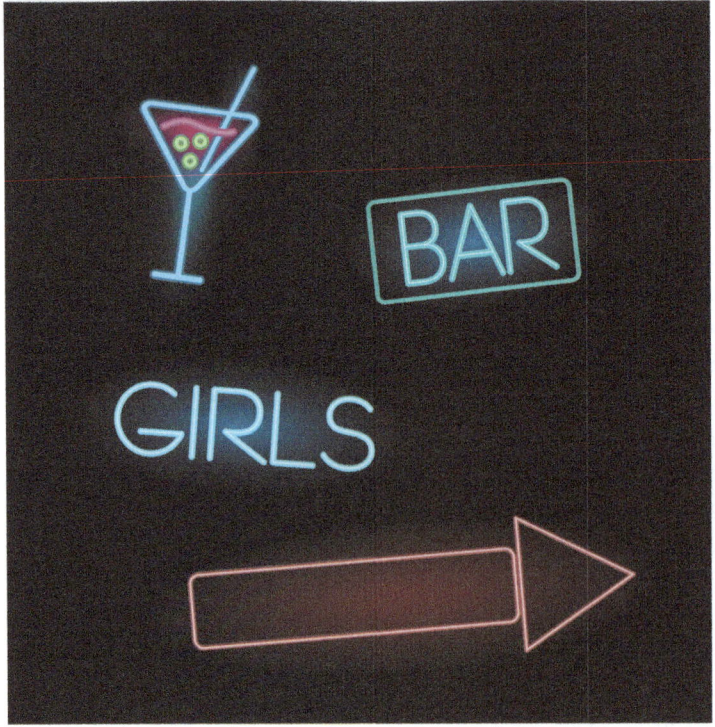

Figure 15.6 Neon Sign

Neon[10]

By Kathryn Cresswell

Bright-shining brilliance
Illuminating pavements
Showing the litter of our ways
Illustrating seediness
Tawdry flashing Motel signage,
Porn Porn Porn
And the neon sign breaks
Just like life.

Songs that mention neon:

Conway Twitty: Rainy Night in Georgia
'. . . Neon signs a-flashin', taxi cabs and buses passin' through the night.'

Pretenders: Night in My Veins
*'He's got me up against the back of a Pick-up truck
Out of sight of the neon and glare'*

Chris Wall: Somewhere Between 40 and Falling Apart
'Neon suits me best.'

Laura Cantrell: Somewhere Some Night
'And somewhere some night, among the neon lights, I'll find my baby.'

Kris Kristopherson: Just the Other Side of Nowhere
'Fadin' from the neon nightime glow here, headin' for the light of day.'

Terry Allen: High Plains Jubilee
'They slow-danced through the neons like sorrow through a song.'

Derailers: Bar Exam
'I'm taking the bar exam under a neon sign. I'm going to graduate when you're off my mind.'

Killers: Neon Tiger
'Run neon tiger there's a lot on your mind.'

Alphaville: Big in Japan
'Neon on my naked skin'

Wayne Hancock: Thunderstorms and Neon Signs
'The warmth of the neon when a bad storm was moving in'

Whiskeytown: Jacksonville Skyline
'Neon signs and car dealerships and islands'

Alan Jackson: Chasin' That Neon Rainbow
'I'm chasin' that neon rainbow, I'm livin' that honkey tonk dream'

Sheryl Crow: Leaving Las Vegas
'Life springs eternal, on a gaudy neon street'

Son Volt: Tear Stained Eye
'Looking for a purpose from a neon sign'

Slaid Cleaves: Drinkin' Days
'No more fights or neon lights.'

Brooks & Dunn: Neon Moon
'I'll be alright as long as there's light from a neon moon'

Neil Young: On Broadway
'They say the neon lights are bright on Broadway'

David Lee Murphy: Party Crowd
'Oh I'm sittin here soakin' up the neon lights, misery looking for some company'

Bob Dylan: Simple Twist of Fate
'Stopped into a strange hotel, With the neon burning bright.'

Randy Travis: The Truth is Lying Next to You
'Don't need a neon moon to make my nights shine.'

Creedence Clearwater Revival: Up Around the Bend
'Where the neon turns to wood.'

John Mayer: Neon
'She's always buzzin' just like neon, neon, neon, neon'

Elton John: In Neon
'In neon the dreams in the light of a promise that dies'

Notwist: Neon Golden
'Neon golden like all the lights.'

Kinks: Underneath the Neon Sign
'Electronic nature made by man with robots in mind.
Big city lights guide my way into the night, darkness shines
When I'm standing underneath the neon sign.'

Merle Haggard: Swinging Doors
'And my new home has got a flashing neon sign'

Handsome Family: All the TVs in Town
'When the air hangs like snakes of the flashing neon signs, it seems like there's nothing along these broken roads, but blinking lights on creaking metal poles. Like a thousand crying eyes dropping tears in the lights of all the TVs in town'

Handsome Family: A Thousand Diamond Rings
'Neon signs above the old motels, warehouse stores and strip malls'

Jude: Charlie Says
'The city gets bright I can't see, The neon lights don't work on me"

Isobel Campbell and Mark Lanegan: Trouble
"When the neon lights that find you. Leave our memory far behind you"

References

1   The circle of four elements is an analysis method taught in depth at The Dynamis School.
2   Ecclesiastes 1.1. Available online at: https://biblia.com/bible/esv/Fc1.1
3   Mark 1:8. Available online at: https://biblia.com/bible/esv/Mk1.8
4   Revelations 3:20. Available online at: https://www.biblegateway.com/passage/?search=Revelation+3%3A20
5   Mistlberger P. T. *Introduction to Psycho-Spiritual Alchemy*. Available online at: http://www.ptmistlberger.com/psychospiritual-alchemy.php.
6   Von Baeyer H. C. (2000). "The Lotus Effect". *The Sciences* 40: 12–15. Available online at: Exerptshttp://www.lotusfertility.com/The_Lotus_Effect_in_Botany_and_Philosophy.html
7   A Tribute to Buddism. Available online at: http://www.jendhamuni.com/lotus-flower-symbol-of-purity-and-great-beauty/
8   Herrick N. *Sacred Plants, Human Voices*. Grass Valley CA: Hahnemann Clinic Publishing, 2003.
9   Lyric by Paul Simon (1964), song performed by Simon and Garfunkel (Columbia Records, 1964) http://www.sglyrics.myrmid.com/sounds.htm
10 http://www.everypoet.net/element/display.php?symbol–Ne.

16

NEON MMM MIASMS

On reaching the MMM potency of perception we touch the collective: miasms.

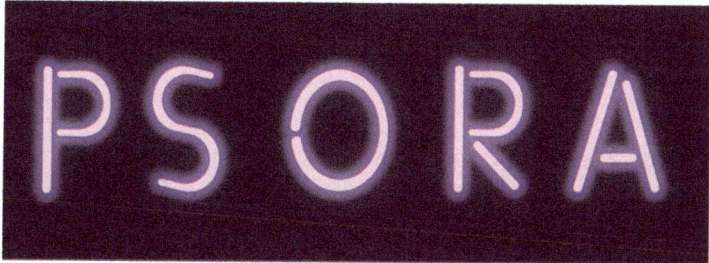

Figure 16.1 *Neon Psora*

As Neon is in the second period it relates to an early stage of psora.

While the first period represents disconnection from the universal soul and the beginning of fragmentation, the second period, including Neon, takes a step further into psora by dividing and splitting us from ourselves. Psora is initiated from this basic divide, the primary split between yin and yang. (Figure 16.2)

The One: pre hydrogen, the whole.

Healthy Life: Whole, Helium, incarnation, first susceptibility, latent psora.

Split: Neon, pregnancy, birth, psora.

We will examine Neon's psoric connection. Psora's main physical affinity is the skin. Itching is prominent in Neon. Once we incarnate, yin and yang split from each other and the skin becomes the barrier that separates each of us from the rest of the world. It is this barrier, the skin firmament, that itches, like a knocking on the door, and we scratch in an attempt to reconnect.

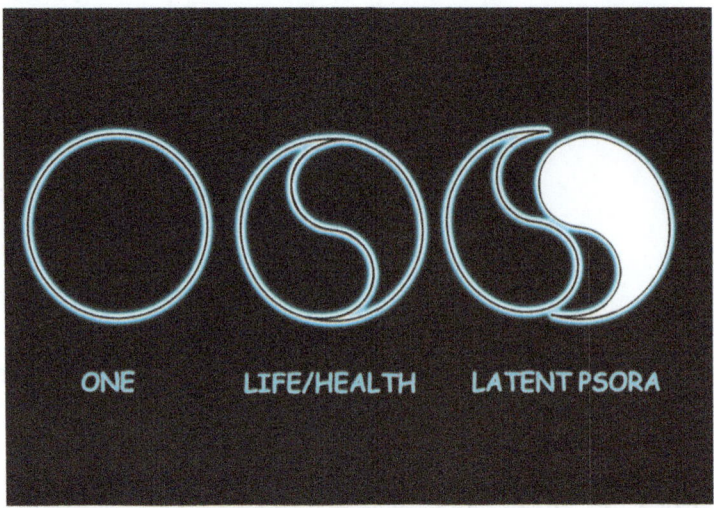

ONE   LIFE/HEALTH   LATENT PSORA

Figure 16.2 Evolution of psora

In *Chronic Diseases*,[1] Hahnemann tells us that psora is contracted the moment the midwife comes into contact with the baby, first touch.

> Yea, often a babe, when being born, is infected while passing through the organs of the mother, who may be infected (as is not infrequently the case) with this disease; or the babe receives this unlucky infection through the hand of the midwife, which has been infected by another parturient woman (or previously); or, again, a suckling may be infected by its nurse, or, while on her arm, by her caresses or the caresses of a strange person with unclean hands.

The moment newborn Neon ventures into the world, it comes into contact with the most infectious miasm of all – psora. Contamination is immediate.

As Hahnemann explains, the slightest contact between two skin surfaces can excite the psoric infection, particularly at birth. As skin contact is the exciting cause of psora, and as an exciting cause is always similar to the underlying chronic susceptibility, skin contact must be a major aspect of latent psora.[2] The touch of two skins is a symbol of our basic psoric delusion, our belief that we are separate from each other; that our skin divides us. In other words, the primary susceptibility of latent psora is the separation of one soul from another as they detach from the united sea of souls.

We meet this primary spilt in Hydrogen and Helium, when they separate from the one. It is only because our incarnated soul is already divided that Neon takes a step further in splitting us from ourselves and others, creating the physical division of skin and firmament. Helium contains the seeds of

TABLE 16.1 Latent psora Helium and psoric Neon

Helium	Neon
Latent Psora	Psora
Souls divided	Skin divided
Line	Surface
Light and dark split	Upper and lower waters split
Day One of creation	Day Two of creation

the potential split, while Neon manifests it in the body. Neon is the acute, relative to Helium's chronic. Table 16.1 illustrates this point.

It is a common mistake to think of psora as an eruption. Rather the archetypical symptom of psora is an itch, more specifically, itch without eruption. This symptom, itch without eruption, appears in the Neon proving. An itch, especially the psoric, voluptuous itch, is a nervous phenomena and not a skin problem. Eruptions appear later as a result of this nervous disturbance. It is for this reason I consider itch without eruption to be one of the most psoric symptoms. This itch represents a deep internal problem, a deviation of the bio-energetic-electromagnetic vital force, as projected through the nerves, and therefore it cannot be treated with ointments or creams as so many allopaths suppose.

In chronic disease the bio-energetic-electromagnetic energy, which we term vital force, changes the direction of its flow, progressing from health towards incurable, auto-immune disease. Scratching or rubbing is a way to generate static electricity or to create a magnetic force, aimed at re-reversing the polarizaton of vital bio-electromagnetic energy. Itching, scratching and rubbing are attempts to generate enough static electricity to reverse its flow. This is a somewhat akin to the action of a magnet moving relative to an electric coil to create a current (Faraday's law of induction). The rubbing is magnetic and the vital force a spiral.

How do we know that our internal electric polarity (or phase) is reversed? There are two factors. The first is that the psoric mirror we live through reverses our whole perception of truth. Hence the very essence of chronic disease is our relentless march in the wrong direction, towards inevitable destruction of the self. The vital force literally gets its wires crossed, which is why Hahnemann now deems it to be stupid (*Organon*[3] § 72). If you doubt this, just look at the world around you.

The second factor indicating the reversal of bio-electric vital flow is sexuality.

The voluptuous nature of the itch, which induces scratching or rubbing, also indicates its relationship to sexuality. Voluptuous itch is literally a primordial sexual stimulation. Both the voluptuous, nervous itch and the sexual act are attempts at reversing the bio-energetic-electromagnetic identity at the core of our being; gender exchange. As sexual energy builds up, our shadow side gradually creeps to the fore, while our restricting consciousness retreats to the posterior. At the same time our physical and mental itch increases, inducing voluptuous scratching and rubbing. The reversal occurs at the point of orgasm, when electrical contraction flips yin back into yang and vice versa, transforming dissatisfaction into bliss. This is followed by relaxation that usually manifests as rolling over in bed; electrical excitement flips to electrical indifference.

The result of skin contact between two individuals is static electricity, the electrical spark of mutual attraction between two opposing electrical poles. We all know this feeling from a brush of skins, an accidental touch at the cinema. This spark is the precursor of both itch and sexual desire, which have the same origin: bio-energetic-electromagnetic currents of two human beings who yearn to reconnect. The underlying issue is that the touch of two skins acts as a reminder that we were once all one being in the common sea of souls. This vital process is absent before incarnation, but appears with the basic spilt of yin and yang in Neon. Itching and sex are a vicarious, but ultimately futile, attempt to regain our lost unity and create an endless cycle of need and gratification, the *'Itchy, scratchy show'*.

Extreme itching of labia. Scratching caused sexual arousal; had to leave the room to do this. Relieved by applying ice or cold water.

It therefore appears that the primal nature of psora is related to gender, sexuality and internal polarity. Let us now examine the polarity issue of Neon in a deeper context.

From Hahnemann's writing it might seem that the infection is simply a result of skin touching skin, the contact with a mother, nurse or midwife. Perhaps a virus jumps across the divide? However, the lightening-like speed of the infection from a mere touch seems strange; a viral infection would not occur that quickly. Rather the nature of the psoric infection is twofold: energetic and psychic. The midwife, long-infected by a psoricly reversed bio-electric charge, need only touch the baby to reverse the direction of their vital flow. This is the nature of induction when two electrified coils come close to each other.

But the touch of skins also symbolises a deeper psychic contamination, for there is nothing that infects faster than the speed of thought; the virus of a concept instantly transferred from one human to another.

All too often the first sentence that a newborn baby and its parents hear is the midwife announcing 'It's a boy' or 'It's a girl'. This is the moment of psoric infection: Welcome to the new world, you are now labelled. This is the primal split into a yin or yang as a fixed, inflexible identity. From this point on the parents will deepen the gender divide by choosing pink dresses, blue shirts, dolls, cooking sets, hammers or guns until the child can express its own desires and tendencies. Identification is one of the roots of psora, and our earliest identification is a gender-based spilt.

In modern times this split occurs in the third month of pregnancy when an ultrasound examination reveals the child's sex, forcing the parents into premature attitudes concerning the foetus's sexual identity. There is no doubt that the mother's preconceptions regarding the child's gender will infect the foetus in utero; psora comes early nowadays.

Once the child is inflicted with an identity, it is infected with psora. Concepts such as I am male, I am female, I am a capitalist or I am an anarchist are the result of one-sided identification. We love our 'one half'' and hate our 'other half'. Even a mere thought can inflict this miasmatic predisposition. If someone whispers 'This person is a liar', it immediately creates love and hate, the 'us and them' effect. The four-part soul is now deeply entrenched in the identity of a one-quarter soul.

Another aspect of Neon's skin affinity is its superficial nature. Like a baby, Neon can be selfish and consumed with skin-deep desires, a two-dimensional personality with no depth. Everything is on the surface.

Dreamt I saw the doctor medicate and peel the entire skin off the back of a child.

Neon's development within the psoric miasm is further illustrated by the time and space issues of this remedy, the inability to be in the here and now. According to quantum physics, time and space are only secondary forces, and the primary force of the universe is entanglement.[4] Helium exists in the primary world where neither space nor time exist, while Neon begins to untangle this entanglement into our linear concept of time.

Psora reverses our perception of the true nature of the universe, distorting it by smoke and mirrors.[i] Why else would humans behave the way they do? Neon is the first mirror, a firmament that obscures the One.

Dream of finding a broad-rimmed hand mirror in a bathroom. I thought it belonged to a girl down the corridor so went to knock on her door. I knocked several times. She didn't answer, though I could see her inside through the keyhole. Eventually she opened the door. A beautiful view over the sea from her balcony window, with two beds and a cot in her room. She said the mirror belonged to somebody in Room 20. I searched up and downstairs and in a different wooden building for room 20; I couldn't find it. So I handed the mirror in at a reception area.

As we descend the periodic table deeper into the miasmatic predicament, there will be more mirrors to come. Perverted psoric perceptions invert everything we see. In a psora-free world, time would flow in reverse, future to past. We would grow younger with each passing day, and not the dreadful reverse.

Dreamt she showed me photos of herself getting progressively younger until she was a baby.

In such a world, the fruit of our life would be the pure bliss of being a baby, rather than the discontent of old age.

By distorting the truth, psora craftily disguises itself, misrepresenting our image of what psora really is. We imagine it to be a dreadful skin disease 'caught' by our ancestors some 10,000 years ago, and passed down through the generations by poor psoric victims. Hence, we can easily blame great, great granddaddy and great grandmamma for our afflictions: 'It wasn't us, and there is nothing we can do about it'!

The truth is that psora happens at one time only, now. At every given moment we can be caught in its web of lies, or transcend for a moment to regain the bliss of truth. The choice is ours, here, now, Neon.

---

[i] For more information on the relationship between nerves, itch and mirrors, please see the following article, Gawande A. The Itch. *New Yorker*, June 30 2008.

Its mysterious power may be a clue to a new theory about brains and bodies.

http://www.newyorker.com/reporting/2008/06/30/080630fa_fact_gawande?current Page=all

Psora

Psora,
As if,
a mite jumped up,
and bit our skin,
infecting human kind,
then generations of suppression,
drove it to our mind,
now microbes and bacteria,
consume our inner being,
while other undesirables,
cause endless misery.
As if from sins of fathers,
and generations gone,
we point accusing finger,
and blame heredity.
Then separating good from bad
in fixed morality,
to love our friends
and hate our foes,
who is the enemy?
As if we had no part to play
in tearing female from her man.
in separating from our heart,
can thought infect?
you know it can!
and now six billion people,
cells of a half dead corpse,
membranes thick as fig leaf,
psoriasis hard and coarse.
We cut our trees, we plant cement,
cloak earth in concrete robe,
rip our mother's atmosfear,
science paves the road.
search in vain for culprit,
the answer lies inside
if we persist in looking
it will persist to hide
the price of knowing is to know,
and knowledge leads to fear,
proliferation, isolation,
gaia sheds a tear.
Psora,
As if.

References

1 Hahnemann CS. *Chronic Diseases* Encyclopedia Homeopathica Archibel Homeopathic Software.

2 Sherr J. *Lectures on Acute and Chronic Disease*, unpublished.

3 Hahnemann CS. *The Organon of the Healing Art* (6th edn). New Delhi: B. Jain Publishers Pvt Ltd, 2003.

4 Vedral V. Living in a Quantum World. *Scientific American*. June, 2011. Available online at: http://www.scientificamerican.com/article.cfm?id=living-in-a-quantum-world

17

ALTERNATIVE DIMENSIONS

In Chapter 10, 'New Dimensions' I discussed the development from line to surface, the evolution from the first dimension of Helium's vertical line to a two-dimensional vertical plane. In this section I will change perspective, and start with the Helium line, oriented horizontally.

My purpose is to explore the analogies between three factors: the noble gases, the dimensions and the days of creation. As far as I know this has never been done before, and I find the correspondences to be fascinating as well as useful in practice.

To understand this correspondence we will have to change our point of view. The first dimension is a line. In the previous chapter I assumed the Helium line to be vertical. We will now rotate the axis by 90°. (Figure 17.1)

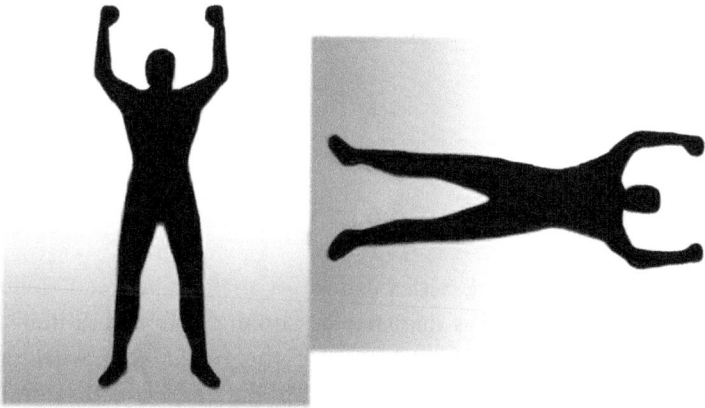

Figure 17.1 *Changing point of view*

It is essential to differentiate between direction (axis) and dimensions. The three directions are height, width and length (Figure 17.2). The three dimensions are line, surface and cube (Figure 17.3) It makes no difference to the dimensions what axis each of the three lines lie on, it is the

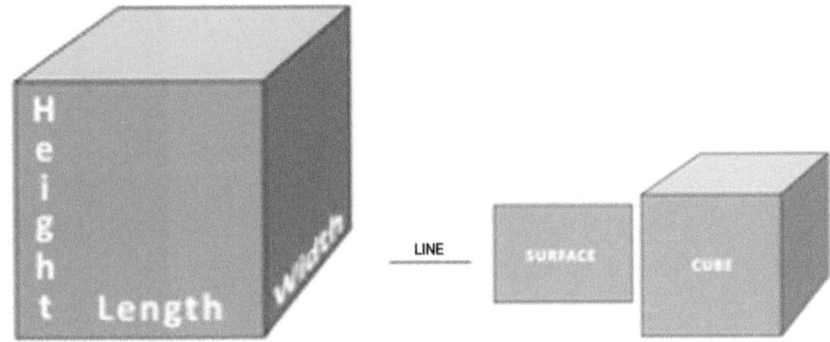

Figure 17.2 *Three directions*   **Figure 17.3** *Three dimensions*

combination of one, two or three lines placed at 90° to each other that forms the first three dimensions.

We now go back to the beginning. Evolution starts with a pre-Hydrogen singularity in which all dimensions are compressed into one (Figure 17.4).

Figure 17.4 *All dimensions in one, singularity*

In the first book of this series I drew an analogy between Helium and the first day of creation as depicted in Lurianic Cabbala. Initially, God's light is everywhere. In order to create the world God withdraws his omnipresent light leaving a void, the initial dark and chaotic world before creation begins. Only one straight line of light penetrates this void, a reminder of God's presence in the world (Figure 17.5). This is analogous to the unfolding of the first dimension, the Helium line of light, the straight line of an un-incarnated individual soul before it tilts into life (Figure.17.6)

While I previously presented the Helium line as vertical, we could equally assume this line to be horizontal. This is just a matter of changing points of view. Such a horizontal line would separate above from below,

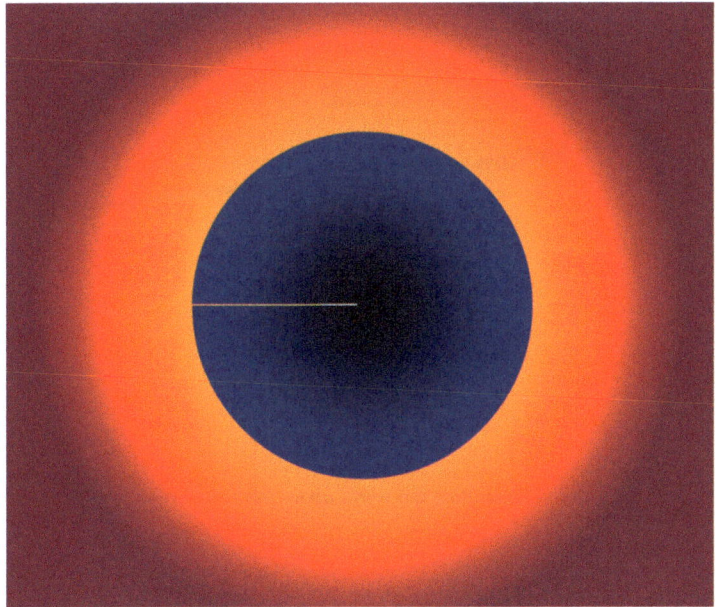

Figure 17.5 God withdraws his light to create the world, leaving one ray

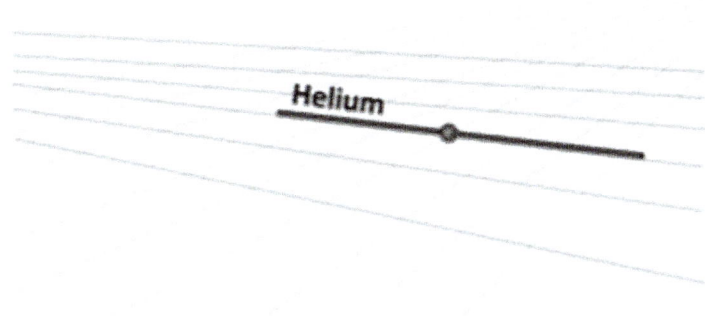

Figure 17.6 Helium unfolding into the first dimension, line

(Figure 17.7) a reflection of the Helium proving, which depicts the separation of the high spiritual world from the lower world of physical manifestation.

Helium is trapped in its line. To free itself, it must split and stretch into a new dimension: surface. It splits into two, horizontally, as it progresses

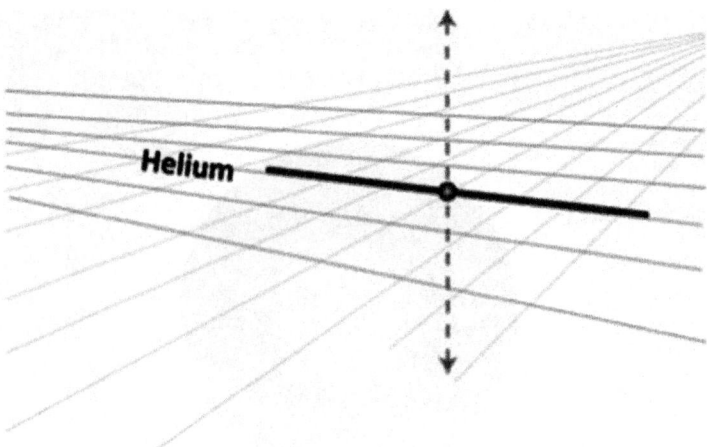

Figure 17.7 Helium's line separating the world above from the world below

through the second period, as well as through the second day of creation (Figure 17.8).

And God said: 'Let there be a firmament in the midst of the waters, and let it divide the waters from the waters.' Genesis 1:6

Once the split has fully manifested, a new direction is created: width (Figure 17.9).

The combination of both of these lines, length and width, creates a two-dimensional surface (Figure 17.10).

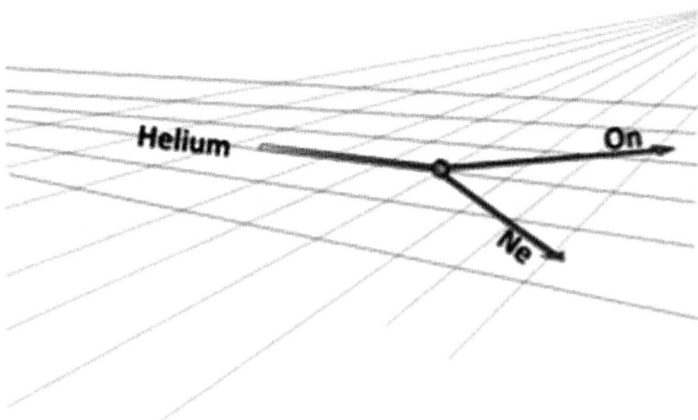

Figure 17.8 Helium's line splitting in two, horizontally

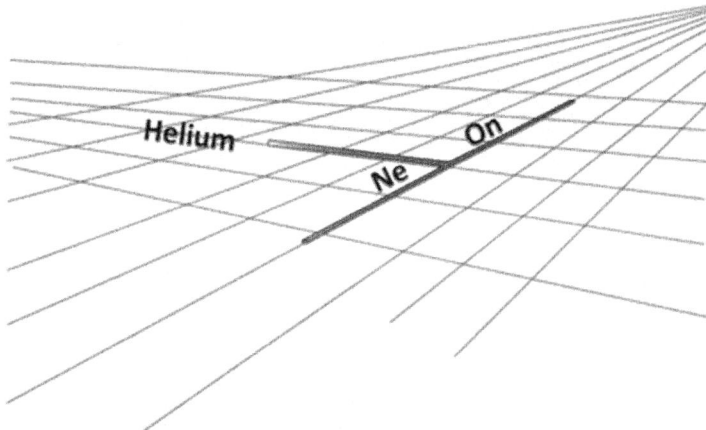

Figure 17.9 *A new perpendicular line manifests within a horizontal plane, creating a second direction*

> And God made the firmament, and divided the waters which were under the firmament from the waters which were above the firmament; and it was so. And God called the firmament Heaven. And there was evening and there was morning, a second day.
>
> Genesis 1:7

The firmament is a surface. Surface allows for bending of shapes. In this second dimension, the straight line of light can curve and swirl, creating the spiral patterns of the galaxies, which Neon longs for (Figure 17.11).

We can thus perceive that on the first day of creation, light or line were created. On the second day, firmament and surface were created. Neon seeks to penetrate this firmament into the third dimension. As we will see

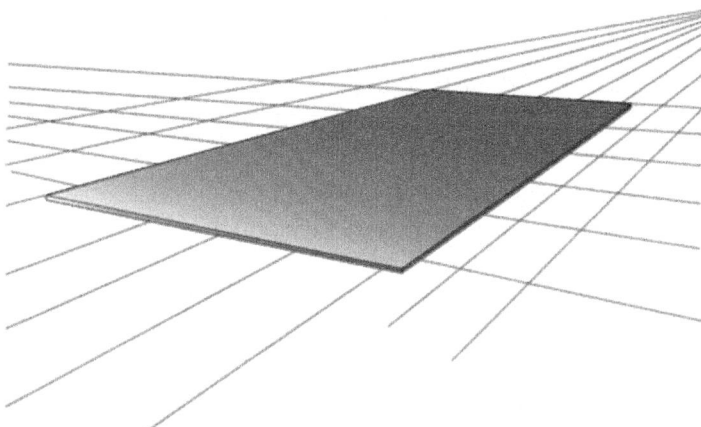

Figure 17.10 *Two perpendicular lines creating a two-dimensional surface*

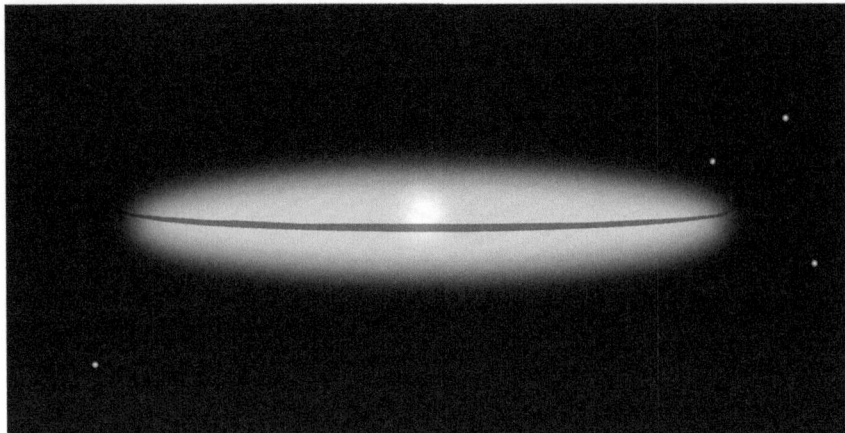

Figure 17.11 Firmament surfaces: Galaxy

the third axis of existence, height, will be created on the third day, giving rise to three-dimensional objects, such as the cube. This process is initiated in the second half of the second day, after the waters recede, exposing fertile earth on which seed and tree and fruit will thrive. Neon strives vertically towards the heavens and adds a third dimension to the world.

Space-time

Here and now: **Helium** for **He**re, **Neon** for **N**ow. We might say that Helium, in the first dimension of line, develops space, while Neon, in the second dimension of surface, evolves time. Thus time is perpendicular to space (Figure 17.9), a theory that is supported by some physicists.[1]

The Helium proving depicts a soul trying to find its place: heaven or earth (see Figure 17.7). There is no time in the world between life and death. Neon depicts a linear time: in its negative side, it splits into future and past. In its positive side, Neon is wholly in the Now, a new-born recreating itself again at every moment, a state of constant bliss.

This analogy might suggest that space could exist before time (Helium before Neon). Mainstream physics rejects this notion as an oxymoron (If it happened *before* then there had to be time). This may be true or it may simply be semantics. There is some debate on this subject. Physics Professor Günter Nimtz has investigated 'tunnelling barriers'. In a series of experiments he demonstrated superluminal velocities, showing that electromagnetic radiation exceeds the speed of light and thus displays a space of zero-time.[2]

In the first paragraph of his book *Eternity: God, Soul, New Physics,* Trevelyan discusses these and other experiments:

> Consider the following propositions. Eternity, the theological construct of space without time, can now be produced in the laboratory. The soul, which has a quantifiable, physical nature, is compatible with Eternity. The physics of time proves that a creator God must be outside of time, bringing time into being with the universe, rather than initiating a universe at a particular point in pre-existing space and time. Are these ideas speculation, fantasy, or science fiction?... No, this is hard-nosed, down-to-earth science: the results of experiments with machines made of metal, glass and electronics.[3]

The model of time as an arrow pointing in one direction is outdated. This uni-directional concept of time is now viewed as the result of limited observation by a particular spectator. Quantum physics dictates that phenomena may occur everywhere and anywhere until they are 'frozen' into one position by observation. Thus we might say that there *is no direction to time.* Everything just exists in a nebulous, a-temporal continuum. Only when something becomes observable does it enter the one-dimensional time continuum.

The arrow of time does not exist in the universe as a whole. It is present solely in individual subjective views of the universe.[4] Individual subjective views appear only once an individual subjective soul manifests. Time exists before Helium, but there is no one to observe and freeze it into a linear arrow. You may recall that Helium sees things in 360° around the head, rather than in a limited, linear fashion. It takes an individual Neon observer to constrict time into a line.

From a physics point of view, these thoughts are in the realm of the speculative. But when we consider the analogy of the periodic table unfolding into the dimensions, and add in the proving data from the remedies, these ideas are at least food for thought. In the space of time we will come to see how Argon develops a third spatial dimension, after which Krypton curves linear time. Rough seas ahead.

References

1   Durgun M. E. Ch 6.2 Time as a Dimension in Space-Time Geometry in *Geometric Generalization of the Structure of Nature.* 2007 http://www.unitytheory.info/time_dimension_spacetime.html

2   Nimtz G. Tunnelling Barriers http://www.popularscience.co.uk/?tag=gunter-nimtz

3   Trevelyan. *Eternity: God, Soul, New Physics,* Amazon Kindle Edition 2013.

4   Goertzel B. On the Physics and Phenomenology of Time. In: *Ben Goertzel's Essays and Papers.* Available online at: http://www.goertzel.org/papers/timepap.html

18

PERIOD II SYNTHESIS

In Neon, the second period completes God's oneness to the power of two. Every noble gas provides an answer to a question posed by the preceding period, while at the same time posing a question to the following period. We yearn to return to the previous period, but are forced to move forward and seek new solutions.

The periodic table of our evolution is a one-way street. Our true home lies behind us, but we are doomed to travel down the road seeking temporary accommodation. A firmament guards the way back, occluding the stars. There is only one way to return to the source, and that is by utilising the 'law of similars' in all its manifestations. The simillimum will align us with the force.

This evolution can be summed up by the following synthesis (based on a vertical orientation of the Helium line).

Pre Creation: I am truly One

Hydrogen: I have lost my oneness.

Helium: Delusion I am one, a line.

Helium pathology: Stuck in a line. Reluctance to lean forward or split.

Helium's question to period two and Neon: How will you deal with my delusion?

Period two and Neon's solution to Helium's delusion of oneness: Divide, splitting line into width. Line combined with width creates a two-dimensional surface.

Neon's pathology: I am two, leaning forward and backward. Stuck in a two-dimensional world and subject to the itch of desire.

Neon's reverse exit strategy: Unite upright and transcend.

Neon's forward exit strategy: Seek a new dimension.

Neon's questions to the third period: How will you deal with my two dimensional division? What is the next dimension?

Trailer: The third period's solution will be found in 'Argon'

19

MOVING ON

In the watery world of Neon everything is always new. There is no past, only motion. Water is always moving, and there is never a point of reference. It seeks its own level, always striving for an even, flat surface. We must either reverse direction towards the homogenous oneness of pre-Hydrogen, or create something permanent in the world. We crave for terra firma to give us a stable base, something we can stand on, a place to build our home and store past memories. We must move on to the third period, natrium to chlorum: Earth.

From

I had thoughts of albatrosses circumnavigating the earth without having to touch the ground.

To

I am all in the now, especially in my lower legs and feet. At last, I touch the earth.

Neon is the bridge between the second and third periods. As well as being the last element of the second period, one might say that Neon is the first element of the third period. This third period represents the flowering of psora, and presents our basic anti-psoric remedies: Natrum, Magnesium, Alumina, Silica, Phosphorus, Chlorum and, of course, Sulphur. Here the new dimensions develop; land into trees, itch into eruption. As we traverse the third period, psora becomes well entrenched.

We have created the barrier, and the barrier is within; we must either dissolve it or learn to live with it. In Neon, we attempt to cure the divide by reuniting back to one line, an *a-lign-ment* with Helium's axis. If we cannot reunite with our twin soul in Helium, the baton will be passed to the next noble. New avenues will open up. The classroom will take place in the third period and the teachers will range from Natrum to Muriaticum. Graduation will take place at Argon. See you there.

Neo-Natal

Neo-Natal
False bright
Light the night,
Divide, unite,
Knock-knock
Stand upright-
Through my window
Much delight
Deep space
Endless might
Or forward bend
Occlude the force
Now I'm longing
for the source,
longing
For the stars so bright
Ovum waiting
For white knight,
Long tailed steed
To plant a seed
Time is flowing
Into need

Still blue
Waters part
Ready? Start.
New life
Itch and strife-
The light is on
What a con
And we are gone
To Ar-gon.

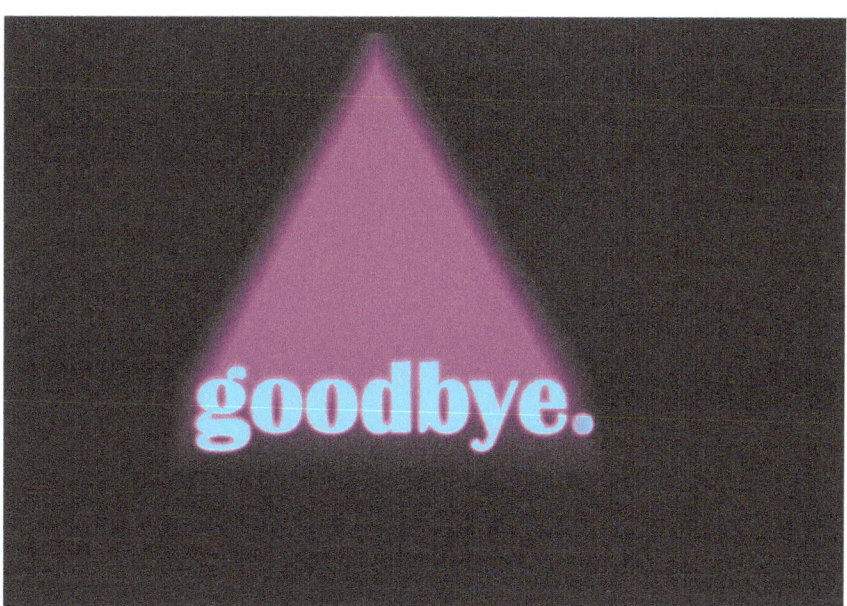

Which came first, neon or water?

The following is my correspondence with Professor Carlo U. Segre – Professor of Physics, Illinois Institute of Technology, via www.allexperts.com

Question:

Dear Sir

Could you please tell me which was created first in the order of cosmological creation of elements and molecules: the element neon or the water molecule?

With thanks

Jeremy

Answer:

Dear Jeremy

You are actually asking about two completely different processes as water is a molecule and Neon is an atom. A better question would be the sequence of creation of Hydrogen, Oxygen, and Neon. Once you have Hydrogen and Oxygen, then formation of water is possible if the temperature is low enough.

In the Big Bang model of the universe, the first thing that is formed after the quark-gluon plasma is no longer stable (that is the universe has cooled down sufficiently) is the hydrogen nucleus (i.e. a proton). When the temperature cools further, electrons bind to the protons to form Hydrogen atoms. The atoms will then condense to form stars which sustain nuclear fusion, creating Neon nuclei and eventually heavier and heavier nuclei (not atoms) inside the stars. When the stars explode in novae and supernovae, even heavier nuclei are formed and dispersed in such a way as is possible to form planets like the Earth.

Therefore, the answer to your question is that Hydrogen is formed first and Oxygen nuclei can be formed inside a star but will not be atoms and will not generally form water until they are expelled from the star and are able to combine with Hydrogen gas. Neon is formed during the stellar explosions.

So, I suppose it is possible to find interstellar water before you might expect to have Neon.

Cheers,

Carlo

Question:

Dear Carlo

Thank you for your very helpful answer. However could you please explain: if the neon ATOM is formed DURING a stellar explosion, and the oxygen ATOM only after it cooled down, why would neon not come first?

Or, If only the neon NUCLEI formed during the explosion, how long would it take to form a neon ATOM. Would that happen before or after oxygen cooled down enough to form an atom and subsequently the water molecule?

Will the oxygen nuclei form before the neon nuclei because they are lighter?

I am interested partly because it seems neon and water have the same number of protons/electrons.

Sorry to be persistent, I appreciate your time and knowledge.

Answer:

Hi Jeremy

Your original question asked about the water MOLECULE, not the oxygen ATOM. If you ask me about oxygen and neon as atoms, then it is likely that oxygen is formed first, since it is possible in the last stages before going nova, a star is actually producing some heavier nuclei in the fusion process. But these are only oxygen nuclei (not even atoms) because in the core of a star, the temperature is sufficiently high that all atoms are completely ionised and there is a plasma of electrons and nuclei. You can see how water has no chance of forming in this environment as a molecule requires the presence of electrons to form bonds. Neon atoms, or rather nuclei, can probably only form after a nova since the atomic number is sufficiently large.

So the answer is that while the combined atomic numbers of H_2O and Ne are the same, inside the core of a star a molecule cannot exist because of the temperature and since the ejection of nuclei from the core of a star requires a nova, then the neon nucleus, and then the atom upon cooling, will form before the temperature is low enough to permit the formation of a molecule such as water.

Carlo

INDEX